Social Media and Youth Mental Health

Social Media and Youth Mental Health

Edited by
Vicki Harrison, M.S.W.
Anne Collier, M.A.
Steven Adelsheim, M.D.

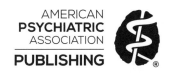

AMERICAN
PSYCHIATRIC
ASSOCIATION
PUBLISHING

If you wish to buy 50 or more copies of the same title, please go to www.appi.org/special-discounts for more information.

Copyright © 2025 American Psychiatric Association Publishing

ALL RIGHTS RESERVED

First Edition

Manufactured in the United States of America on acid-free paper
28 27 26 25 24   5 4 3 2 1

American Psychiatric Association Publishing
800 Maine Avenue SW, Suite 900
Washington, DC 20024-2812
www.appi.org

Library of Congress Cataloging-in-Publication Data
Names: Harrison, Vicki, 1972- editor. | Collier, Anne (Writer and youth advocate) editor. | Adelsheim, Steven, editor. | American Psychiatric Association Publishing, issuing body.
Title: Social media and youth mental health / edited by Vicki Harrison, Anne Collier, Steven Adelsheim.
Other titles: Social media and youth mental health (Harrison)
Description: First edition. | Washington, D.C. : American Psychiatric Association Publishing, [2024] | Includes bibliographical references and index.
Identifiers: LCCN 2024004324 (print) | LCCN 2024004325 (ebook) | ISBN 9781615375011 (paperback : alk. paper) | ISBN 9781615375028 (ebook)
Subjects: MESH: Social Media | Psychology, Adolescent | Media Exposure | Mental Disorders | Psychology, Child | Young Adult
Classification: LCC RJ503 (print) | LCC RJ503 (ebook) | NLM WS 462.5.T4 | DDC 616.8900835--dc23/eng/20240213
LC record available at https://lccn.loc.gov/2024004324
LC ebook record available at https://lccn.loc.gov/2024004325

British Library Cataloguing in Publication Data
A CIP record is available from the British Library.

Contents

Part I
Foundational

Part II
Clinical Considerations and Special Populations

Contributors

Steven Adelsheim, M.D.
Clinical Professor, Department of Psychiatry and Behavioral Sciences, Stanford University, Stanford, California

Faith Arimoro, M.P.H.
Medical Student, Perelman School of Medicine, University of Pennsylvania, Philadelphia, Pennsylvania

Eleanor Bailey, Ph.D.
Research Fellow, Orygen; Centre for Youth Mental Health, The University of Melbourne, Parkville, Victoria, Australia

Amanda R. Barrett, B.S.
Doctoral student, Department of Educational Psychology, University of Nebraska–Lincoln, Lincoln, Nebraska

Susanne Baumgartner, Ph.D.
Associate Professor, Amsterdam School of Communication Research, University of Amsterdam, The Netherlands

Justine Bautista, M.A.
School of Social Ecology, University of California, Irvine

Sherry Bell, B.A.
Postdoctoral scholar, University of Oregon, Eugene, Oregon

David S. Bickham, Ph.D.
Research Director, Digital Wellness Lab, Boston Children's Hospital; Assistant Professor of Pediatrics, Harvard Medical School, Boston, Massachusetts

Kelly Boudreau, Ph.D.
Associate Professor in Interactive Media Theory and Design, Interactive Media Program, Harrisburg University of Science and Technology, Pennsylvania

Dalton Bourke, M.D.
Clinical Fellow, Clinic for Interactive Media and Internet Disorders, Division of Adolescent/Young Adult Medicine, Boston Children's Hospital and Harvard Medical School, Boston, Massachusetts

Catherine M. Carney, M.A.
Doctoral candidate, Department of Educational Psychology, University of Nebraska–Lincoln, Lincoln, Nebraska

Michael Carter, Ph.D.
Postdoctoral Research Fellow, Digital Wellness Lab, Boston Children's Hospital and Harvard Medical School, Boston, Massachusetts

Linda Charmaraman, Ph.D.
Senior Research Scientist, Youth, Media, and Wellbeing Research Lab, Wellesley Centers for Women, Wellesley College, Wellesley, Massachusetts

Sophia Choukas-Bradley, Ph.D.
Assistant Professor, Teen and Young Adult Lab, Department of Psychology, University of Pittsburgh, Pittsburgh, Pennsylvania

Anne Collier, M.A.
Founder and Executive Director, The Net Safety Collaborative, Salt Lake City, Utah

Allegra R. Gordon, Sc.D., M.P.H.
Assistant Professor, Department of Community Health Sciences, Boston University, Boston, Massachusetts

Jeffrey T. Hancock, Ph.D.
Harry and Norman Chandler Professor of Communication, Department of Communication, Stanford University, Stanford, California

Vicki Harrison, M.S.W.
Program Director, Center for Youth Mental Health and Wellbeing, Department of Psychiatry and Behavioral Sciences, Stanford University School of Medicine, Stanford, California

Emily Izenman, B.A.
Clinical Research Specialist, Digital Wellness Lab, Boston Children's Hospital, Boston, Massachusetts

Rachel Kowert, Ph.D.
Research Director, Take This, Inc., Kirkland, Washington

Kaylee P. Kruzan, Ph.D., L.S.W.
Department of Preventive Medicine, Northwestern University, Chicago, Illinois

Louise La Sala, Ph.D.
Research Fellow, Orygen; Centre for Youth Mental Health, The University of Melbourne, Parkville, Victoria, Australia

Angela Y. Lee, M.A.
Doctoral candidate, Department of Communication, Stanford University, Stanford, California

Sunny X. Liu, Ph.D.
Director of Research, Social Media Lab, Department of Communication, Stanford University, Stanford, California

Chelly Maes, Ph.D.
Postdoctoral Researcher, Leuven School for Mass Communication Research KU, Leuven, Belgium

Ellen Middaugh, Ph.D.
Assistant Professor of Child and Adolescent Development, Lurie College of Education, San Jose State University, San Jose, California

Fatima Bilal Motiwala, M.D.
Clinical Fellow, Clinic for Interactive Media and Internet Disorders, Division of Adolescent/Young Adult Medicine, Boston Children's Hospital and Harvard Medical School, Boston, Massachusetts

Jared S. Noetzel, M.A.
Doctoral student, Department of Educational Psychology, University of Nebraska–Lincoln, Lincoln, Nebraska

Cătălina Maria Popoviciu, M.A.
Doctoral candidate, University of Bucharest, Bucharest, Romania

Michael Rich, M.D., M.P.H.
Founder and Director, Digital Wellness Lab, and Director of the Center on Media and Child Health, Clinic for Interactive Media and Internet Disorders, Division of Adolescent/Young Adult Medicine, Boston Children's Hospital; Associate Professor, Harvard Medical School, Boston, Massachusetts

Savannah R. Roberts, M.A.
Doctoral candidate, Teen and Young Adult Lab, Department of Psychology, University of Pittsburgh, Pittsburgh, Pennsylvania

Jo Robinson, Ph.D.
Professor and Head of Suicide Research, Orygen; Centre for Youth Mental Health, The University of Melbourne, Parkville, Victoria, Australia

Lara Schreurs, Ph.D.
Postdoctoral researcher, School for Mass Communication Research, Faculty of Social Sciences, KU Leuven, Leuven, Belgium

Stephen M. Schueller, Ph.D.
School of Social Ecology, Department of Psychological Science, and Department of Informatics, University of California, Irvine

Valerie Steeves, J.D., Ph.D.
Full Professor, Department of Criminology, University of Ottawa, Ottawa, Ontario, Canada

Jessica Stone, Ph.D.
Chief Executive Officer, Virtual Sandtray, L.L.C., Fruita, Colorado

Susan M. Swearer, Ph.D., L.P.
Willa Cather Professor of Educational Psychology and Chair, Department of Educational Psychology; Professor and Licensed Psychologist, School Psychology Program, University of Nebraska–Lincoln, Lincoln, Nebraska

Amanda Third, Ph.D.
Professorial Research Fellow and Co-Director, Young and Resilient Research Centre, Institute for Culture and Society, Western Sydney University, Sydney, Australia

Michael Tsappis, M.D.
Psychiatrist, Digital Wellness Lab, Boston Children's Hospital; Co-Director, Clinic for Interactive Media and Internet Disorders, Division of Adolescent/ Young Adult Medicine, Boston Children's Hospital; Instructor of Psychiatry, Harvard Medical School, Boston, Massachusetts

Wisnu Wiradhany, Ph.D.
Faculty of Psychology, Atma Jaya Catholic University of Indonesia, Jakarta, Indonesia

Zhiying Yue, Ph.D.
Postdoctoral Research Fellow, Digital Wellness Lab, Boston Children's Hospital and Harvard Medical School, Boston, Massachusetts

Disclosures

The following contributors to this book have indicated a financial interest in or other affiliation with a commercial supporter, a manufacturer of a commercial product, a provider of a commercial service, a nongovernmental organization, and/or a government agency, as listed below:

David S. Bickham, Ph.D. *Advisory Board:* Google, Inc.

Michael Carter, Ph.D. *Employee:* Digital Wellness Lab.

Linda Charmaraman, Ph.D. *Consultant:* Jed Foundation, Meta.

Allegra R. Gordon, Sc.D., M.P.H. *Research Consultant:* Ernst & Young.

Vicki Harrison, M.S.W. *Content Advisory Council:* TikTok (U.S.).

Stephen M. Schueller, Ph.D. *Consultant:* Otsuka Pharmaceuticals; *Scientific Advisory Board:* Headspace Health.

The following contributors had no competing interests to declare:
Steven Adelsheim, M.D.; Faith Arimoro, M.P.H.; Eleanor Bailey, Ph.D.; Amanda R. Barrett, B.S.; Susanne Baumgartner, Ph.D.; Justine Bautista, M.A.; Sherry Bell, B.A.; Kelly Boudreau, Ph.D.; Dalton Bourke, M.D.; Catherine M. Carney, M.A.; Sophia Choukas-Bradley, Ph.D.; Anne Collier, M.A.; Jeffrey T. Hancock, Ph.D.; Emily Izenman, B.A.; Rachel Kowert, Ph.D.; Kaylee P. Kruzan, Ph.D., L.S.W.; Louise La Sala, Ph.D.; Angela Y. Lee, M.A.; Sunny X. Liu, Ph.D.; Chelly Maes, Ph.D.; Ellen Middaugh, Ph.D.; Fatima Bi-

lal Motiwala, M.D.; Jared S. Noetzel, M.A.; Cătălina Maria Popoviciu, M.A.; Michael Rich, M.D., M.P.H.; Savannah R. Roberts, M.A.; Jo Robinson, Ph.D.; Lara Schreurs, Ph.D.; Valerie Steeves, J.D., Ph.D.; Jessica Stone, Ph.D.; Susan M. Swearer, Ph.D., L.P.A; Amanda Third, Ph.D.; Wisnu Wiradhany, Ph.D.; Zhiying Yue, Ph.D.

Introduction

Technological development moves fast and seems to be accelerating. As we write this, both social media and young people's uses of it are changing. Generative artificial intelligence (AI) and chatbots stole the spotlight away from "the metaverse," heating up competition and challenging us all anew. Twitter became "X" and went down a rabbit hole of its own making. In just a few years, video shorts on TikTok, YouTube, and Instagram have had a noticeable impact on how people all over the world interact with media, giving new meaning to "mass media" and changing the way we thought about "social media" just a few years ago. Now, younger generations are using terms such as "opinion fatigue," "social media breaks," and "tricking the algorithm."

All of this brings new energy to a question societies have now been asking for more than 20 years: How do these new kinds of media and technology, with their rapid pace of development, affect the people who use them, who individually and collectively evolve and adapt much more slowly?

We have seen messages from the U.S. Surgeon General, policymakers, and the news media about a mental health crisis among American youth, along with claims that social media is the source of the problem. Although concern about the role of social media in young people's mental health has increased, reaching a fever pitch during the coronavirus disease 2019 (COVID-19) lockdown, most analyses have relied on correlations and focused on individual impacts. To date, few published works have taken a comprehensive, public health view of this issue. Many research studies investigate a particular sliver of effects, usually negative ones, and popular books covering this topic are often directed at parents, offering individual-level coping strategies rather than broader systems recommendations. We have noted a lack of a perspective that considers the impact of our interactions with social media at a societal scale. Yet when we look at the ways in which social media technologies have taken shape, been promoted, used, and incorporated into our lives, we see impacts both on individual experiences and on social groups and society as a whole that can be health-promoting as well as health-eroding. It is not too late to learn from these findings, listen to young people, and change course where needed.

Some of the data that highlight associations between social media and mental health surface caveats that the correlated findings might be more substantial for "vulnerable" people or those with mental health conditions. However, *vulnerability* is not a descriptor that is universally defined, and it begs further inquiry. Collectively, we need more clarity on where the threshold lies between helpful and harmful in social media interactions, acknowledging that it is likely different for different individuals and communities, as the chapters in this book illustrate.

As multiple states and the U.S. Congress begin to pass laws around social media use by minors nearly 20 years into this media era, it appears we are still at the beginning of a process that will take many years to settle out. We hope this book and the other research and debate that are still needed will contribute to sound policy that supports a positive relationship between social media and the mental health, well-being, and privacy of our nation's youth. We feel strongly that young people's meaningful input is essential to policymaking that affects their lives, online and offline, and that their lived experience with technology is needed expertise for research, policymaking, and public discussion.

Through contributions from academic experts as well as the voices of young people, this compilation demonstrates the monumental influence new media has come to have in all aspects of those young lives and summarizes the latest research findings on more than a dozen different aspects of social media as they relate to youth mental health. The book is divided into two sections: Part 1 looks at youth and media use through multiple lenses of adolescent development, and Part 2 considers social media's clinical applications and implications for youth. Through a public health lens, we aim to deliver a comprehensive look at the impact of social media on the mental health of young people today and offer a foundational framework from which mental health professionals, policymakers, industry leaders, and researchers can consider a renewed phase of media innovation that puts health and well-being first and foremost.

We close the book with a chapter rich in youth perspectives on agency because any book considering the relationship between social media and youth mental health must 1) look forward at the potential digital world that youth could inhabit if we were to prioritize the agency, well-being, rights, and lived experience of our current and upcoming generations; 2) challenge proposed solutions (whether they be laws, parental controls, or monitoring software) that jeopardize young people's developmentally appropriate need for agency; and 3) honor the rights of youth—as established in the 30-plus-year-old United Nations Convention on the Rights of the Child—to participation, provision, and protection.

It is our hope that, in concluding the book this way, our readers will be inspired to join or even collaborate with us and many others in cocreating policy, products, and practice with youth—including policymaking and design that prioritizes their well-being, self-efficacy, and human rights in digital spaces that respect, uplift, inform, inspire, and connect us all, providing support and healing where needed.

Vicki Harrison, M.S.W.
Anne Collier, M.A.
Steven Adelsheim, M.D.

Notes From the Editors

On Definitions

Each chapter author(s) uses their own (and sometimes slightly different) definitions of the terms for the population we are discussing, including *youth*, *young people*, and *children and adolescents*. In most instances, authors are referring generally to the ages between roughly 10 and 25 years, when significant social and developmental growth occurs and when social media use increases in frequency and importance, despite the awareness that youth are engaging with forms of social media at even younger ages.

Social media as a term is treated as a singular noun and is a broad classification that will be specifically defined by authors in some of the chapters but on the whole refers to networked digital spaces in which social interaction occurs. We mean "social media" in its broadest sense, zooming out from the narrow analogy of platforms overly focused on the performative aspect of digital social tools, and inclusive of the many types of digital spaces in which youth interactions are happening, including games, end-to-end encrypted chat, Minecraft and Discord servers, one-to-one direct messaging, and group texting. As social media approaches an inflection point, with growing public discontent and regulatory pressure, we cannot know what young people's digital social ecosystem will look like when this book comes out; many aspects will be the same, but not all. We can know that digital social environments are now an ingrained form of "place" and culture in which adolescent sociality and development play out in real time, every day.

Youth Perspectives

It was important to us to include the voices of youth in a body of work that considers their well-being. In the chapters that follow are direct quotes from youth that are intended to help bring some of the concepts to life. The quotes include the participant's age, sex/gender, and name if such details were available. Some names have been modified to protect privacy, some are anonymous, and some are taken directly from conversations, group discussions, or interviews that the chapter authors held with youth.

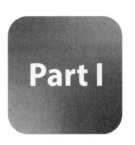

Foundational

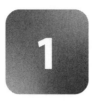

Media's Prominence in the Lives of Youth

Vicki Harrison, M.S.W.

Few would disagree that media plays a prominent role in our lives in the twenty-first century, particularly the daily lives of young people, yet the extent of that influence is debated and possibly underestimated. With the explosion of new media and its instantaneous nature, media is an omnipresent force in the lives of youth today, more than in any prior generation. Among many other things, youth rely on media to understand the world, observe human behavior, and absorb norms. But their developing brains and limited life experience can sometimes leave them vulnerable to various pitfalls that we are still grappling with as a culture. In this chapter I consider some of the challenges and opportunities associated with the evolution and dominance of social media in the lives of youth, highlighting new opportunities for them to accrue various forms of capital and to engage in identity formation and peer relationships, while also taking into account their developmental vulnerabilities, mental health-related risks, and how social media features and norms can sometimes heighten these.

> Social media is both our generation's first encounter with news and our mentor on how to live and grow up.
> —*Edward, age 17*

Media Embedded in All Spheres of Daily Life

Mass media refers to media of all forms (e.g., print, radio, television, magazines) that is transmitted to a large swath of the population in one direction, from producer to consumer. In the late twentieth century, this evolved into *new media*, which is largely internet-based and produced and transmitted in multiple directions by individuals, groups, and organizations. New media (which includes social media) is pervasive around much of the globe in the twenty-first century and is continuously accessible to nearly two-thirds of the global population (Datareportal 2023). Through text, images, sound, and video, its messages serve multiple purposes (i.e., to inform, educate, entertain, and persuade) and are reflective of popular culture in societies worldwide. All types and sources of media express values and social norms, reinforcing them, challenging them, and playing them out in storylines and headlines. Media's influence can be highly positive and educational, but it can also be confusing, disturbing, overwhelming, and sometimes harmful.

Much of the established literature on media's influence has analyzed traditional forms of media (i.e., television and film); however, in recent years, there has been a noticeable spike in literature reviews considering the effects of social media use on adolescent mental health (Valkenburg et al. 2022). Although more inquiry is needed to assess the beneficial and worrying influences of new media on our lives, impacts appear to exist. Yet the associations that have been observed thus far are inconsistent and likely highly dependent on how media use is uniquely intertwined within one's life (Orben 2020). We are no longer passive, occasional viewers, and our experiences in social media and the media ecosystem are constantly evolving and irreversibly embedded in most spheres of our daily lives.

Whereas in prior generations the bulk of mass media was generated by a select few (e.g., journalists, writers, producers, or artists) through a combination of earned credentials and experience, social media platforms invite "user-generated content" from everybody. This not only encourages but relies on users creating and posting content that can in turn be monetized by the platforms, such as through the sale of advertising or product placement, and by the users themselves. Traditional media outlets offered key sources of news, information, and entertainment by established experts, and the absorption of these products was mostly passive—we were media consumers. In the new social media ecosystem, empowering youth and adults to be content creators opens up vast possibilities for self-exploration, skills development, and agency. However, the boundaries between for-profit, educational, and recreational functions are becoming increasingly blurred, rendering social media interactions more complex than mere entertainment or information-seeking.

According to Lombana-Bermudez et al. (2020), youth activities on social media can be viewed as mechanisms by which they can accumulate primary forms of intersecting capital (social, cultural, and economic). For instance, accumulation of likes, follows, and connections (social capital), coupled with creating appealing and contemporary content (cultural capital), can invite monetization possibilities (economic capital) on social media platforms. Although such novel opportunities can be highly empowering and beneficial for youth, they must be balanced with the potential risks, including exploitation, surveillance, limits to privacy, and the potential for burnout (Reidy 2022), associated with the pressure of producing a steady stream of content for one's followers and sponsors.

Social media offers young people a daily range of pursuits, including entertainment, social connection, news, leisure, exploration, community, social status, and profit (Ito et al. 2018). Its use has become more of a necessity than an option in the eyes of many. A remarkable 35% of young people say they use one of the top five social media platforms "almost constantly" (Vogels et al. 2022). As Weinstein and James (2022) described, based on their extensive interviews with teenagers, "in years past—when social technologies supplemented teens' lives but didn't necessarily dictate their every move—avoidance may have been a viable option. Complete and prolonged disconnection just isn't feasible for today's teens when these technologies are essential to their everyday lives, jobs, and school" (p. 91). Yet the relationship young people have with digital platforms has become paradoxical—and some argue inequitable—in that youth are given myriad opportunities to explore, produce, and develop, but, at the same time, their creative and social expressions are lucrative for platforms profiting from their engagement and data (Lombana-Bermudez et al. 2020). With social media integrating into more and more aspects of daily life, opportunities abound to align youth's developmental needs and expectations with the media they engage with in order to avoid the paradox of supporting personal exploration while simultaneously exploiting it for profit.

I use social media for a variety of purposes: I stay in contact with some friends through viewing their posts on social media and...to chat with them. Social media is also my main source of information when it comes to pop culture and style trends. Additionally, I find myself gravitating to

> social media when I am bored, since I know that I can find
> interesting or funny content within seconds.
>   —*Sonia, age 17*

Technology is increasingly being integrated into school classrooms, including platforms and devices with messaging, creating, and collaborating features. The newer "ed tech" (educational technology) products mostly operate apart from the social media platforms most young people engage with outside of school. Many schools are still grappling with how to minimize distractions and other complications (e.g., sexting, cyberbullying, and engaging with noneducational media during class time) associated with students using personal cellular phones or laptops at school, including banning personal devices on campus. Although it is challenging for school policies to keep pace with young people's rapid adoption of new technologies and platforms, it is apparent that blending the two worlds is necessary. Understanding and accepting social media's prominence in the lives of their students will enable educators to cocreate with young people as collaborators in finding productive ways to incorporate dynamic media spaces into educational settings (Goodyear and Armour 2021) and will enable school personnel to engage in proactive education and policy development to address media-based trends that impact education and well-being (Giordano et al. 2022). With media literacy education more important than ever and often delivered through schools, having educators adopt a more collaborative and less resistant approach to social media use will be important for skill development to take hold.

Theories of Media Influence

The influence and interaction of individuals with media is complex and multifaceted. There are several theoretical explanations for the influential interplay between young people and media. These include Bandura's social cognitive theory (formerly social learning theory) that individuals learn by observing behaviors modeled by others and Vygotsky's sociocultural theory that the social and cultural observations and interactions one has with others form the foundation of development (Tudge and Winterhoff 1993). As such, Wartella et al. (2016) suggested that media can afford opportunities for young people to learn and grow beyond their developmental stages and that interactive social media presents a profound opportunity for scaffolded learning, skill development, and growth. They argued that "media and interactive technology have pervasive influence on development and learning and may have the power to influence our values and conceptions of adulthood; namely, priorities, expectations around relationships with others, and definitions of success" (p. 18).

Social comparison theory posits that people compare themselves with others, particularly those similar to themselves, in order to understand their own lives and social standing in the world. For example, some research indicates that exposure to highly idealized images from peers on social media may be more damaging than traditional media images because the peer images are more relatable and closer in social proximity (Fardouly et al. 2017). With media that is by its very definition social in nature, the effects of social learning are likely to be even more pronounced. Use of media occurs within the context of an individual's full life circumstances—where they live, their psychosocial development, their social and family contexts, their prior life experiences, and their cultural identities—which calls for viewing media as one of several interconnected factors in socialization, albeit a powerful one (Paus-Hasebrink et al. 2019).

Media and Social Norms

The messaging, influences, and social scripts communicated through media form the dominant narratives of our culture. Young people's use of media exposes them to values and offers a playbook by which they absorb social norms. In addition to a multitude of learning environments, media can offer a bounty of opportunities for learning and creativity and can inspire empathy, connection, and aspiration by exposing youth to a wide variety of people and experiences different from themselves and their own experiences. According to H. Peyton Young (2015), social norms are "unwritten codes and informal understandings that define what we expect of other people and what they expect of us" (p. 360). Norms enforce themselves because people want to conform to them out of impulses to be part of a group and follow the lead of others and/or out of fear of being sanctioned.

> On social media, "thinspiration" and losing weight is idolized—even normalized. It took me years to realize that what I was doing to my body was dangerous and accept that the world I grew up in was one in which my body dysmorphia and disordered eating was glorified—but not in my best interest.
>
> —*Edward, age 17*

Studies on the introduction of television to an indigenous community in Fiji offered a unique opportunity to demonstrate the influence of media on values and social norms. Three years after the introduction of television in the late 1990s, adolescent girls in that region reported redefined body image ideals more consistent with Western standards and signs of disordered eating, including "the beginnings of weight and body shape preoccupation, purging behavior to control weight, and body disparagement" (Becker 2004, p. 533). A follow-up study by Becker et al. (2011) with this same Fijian population found that indirect media exposure through social networks (the media intake of friends and parents) was just as influential and potentially even more so than a young girl's direct media intake. These results support the theory that effects of media exposure are more multifaceted than content or direct exposure singularly (Bryant and Oliver 2008; Paus-Hasebrink et al. 2019). If media's effects can be mediated (whether positively or negatively) by social and peer factors, this portends to be highly relevant to understanding the potential health impacts of social media environments. Although this will be challenging to study, more inquiry is needed.

Evidence suggests that norms are formed by perception, regardless of whether that perception is accurate. This can lead to friend groups sharing similar social media behaviors and to adolescents' perceptions of how much their peers use social media being associated with their own frequency of use (Marino et al. 2020). Misperceptions can contribute to increases in behaviors that youth perceive to be common or typical. For example, Perkins et al. (2011) suggested that those who engage in a problematic behavior such as bullying may do so feeling a "false majority pressure" and that those who are opposed to the behavior might not speak out against it, thinking their opposition is a minority opinion. Reducing misperceptions and increasing understanding about the actual prevalence of healthy behaviors can subsequently be a strategy employed to increase those behaviors.

Like television, social media is a highly visual medium that, especially among young people, relies heavily on body-centric photograph- or video-based image-sharing, thereby automatically objectifying its users and placing a heavy emphasis on photography and visual expressions of beauty and enjoyment (e.g., selfies and makeovers). In addition to body image, correlations have been explored with regard to media's influence on aggression, substance use, expressions of sexuality, gender roles, and racial stereotypes, among other topics. The effects of media violence on offline behavior have been explored for many years, including more recent questions as to how the conclusions of prior studies apply to new forms of media, such as social media and gaming. Previous work has established a link between media violence and increases in aggressive behaviors in children, and it has raised concerns about desensitizing viewers to acts of violence and normalizing violence as an acceptable response within various, commonly portrayed social scenarios (Anderson et al. 2003). Other studies have established very little positive correlation between violent video gaming and offline violent behavior (Przybylski and Weinstein 2019). Such mixed conclusions serve as a reminder of the complexity involved in understanding media's influence.

Adolescents' exposure to and engagement with pornography, which is commonly accessible via the internet (Thurman and Obster 2021), is another area that has received study regarding its potential purveyance of social norms, including influencing the "sexual scripts" that its viewers adopt (Giordano et al. 2022). In a 2023 report by Common Sense Media, nearly three out of four teenagers reported being exposed to pornography online, with more than half saying they had encountered pornography accidentally. Half of the teens responding indicated that they had seen "violent and/or aggressive pornography, including media that depicts what appears to be rape, choking, or someone in pain" (Robb and Mann 2023, p. 9). The teens reported that they were learning about sex from the material they interacted with. Exposure to pornography has been linked to aggression, permissive sexual attitudes, dominant sexual behaviors, and sexual objectification of oneself and others, raising some concerns about how the sex-related media that young people consume may negatively influence their sexual attitudes, behaviors, and relationships (Grubbs and Kraus 2021).

Furthermore, the reliance of social media platforms on algorithms that track online interactions and clicks in order to personalize one's experience and serve tailored content, including advertising, can skew a user's perception of which social norms are predominant and how they are perceived. As Radesky et al. (2020) wrote, "previous online behaviors shape what is delivered to users via news, notifications, and social media feeds, creating a filter bubble in which all input, unbeknownst to users, is tailored to their interests and creates false norms that can undermine healthy behaviors" (p. 3). Thus, it appears possible media can have a distorted "normative" effect, conveying norms and conventions regardless of whether they are widely accepted.

Unique Considerations of the Adolescent Brain

The span from preadolescence through young adulthood (from approximately ages 12 to 25 years) is a period marked by extraordinary changes within the brain. Heightened attunement to peer influence, risk-taking, impulsivity, sensation-seeking, and exploration are all characteristics of this

pivotal phase of development (Tibber and Silver 2022). Many see this powerful period of brain maturation as a vulnerable time when young people are
highly susceptible to media's positive and negative effects. This reality has
spurred inquiry into the persuasive effects of the advertising young people
encounter via media and has informed policy actions aimed at protecting
them. In 2020, the American Academy of Pediatrics issued a policy statement
titled "Digital Advertising to Children" that expressed concern about tracking
the behaviors of children in order to target them for marketing campaigns because children may lack the abstract thinking skills or impulse control to recognize and resist such campaigns (Radesky et al. 2020). As they explained,

> children are uniquely vulnerable to the persuasive effects of advertising
> because of immature critical thinking skills and impulse inhibition.
> School-aged children and teenagers may be able to recognize advertising
> but often are not able to resist it when it is embedded within trusted social
> networks, encouraged by celebrity influencers, or delivered next to per-
> sonalized content.

During adolescence, the influence of peers and desire for peer acceptance peaks (Elmore et al. 2017). Adolescents are particularly aware of their
peers' thoughts and actions (Telzer et al. 2022) and leverage media to build
connection and community. The internet and social media platforms offer
ripe environments in which peer interactions and peer subcultures (a shared
interest in a common topic, celebrity, or media genre) can be explored and
asserted (Lim 2013). As Lim (2013) explained, "young people incorporate
media content into their peer interactions and appropriate a variety of communication platforms to socialize with their peers, thus generating distinc-
tive traits, norms, practices, codes, and shared identities that make up their
unique peer culture(s)" (p. 322). The anonymity many online spaces offer
allows adolescents to venture into potentially risky subcultures and peer interactions, but the effect of peer influence during adolescence cuts both
ways, meaning the potential for positive, prosocial peer influences is also
heightened (Telzer et al. 2022).

Work by Elmore et al. (2017) suggested that media can act as a "super
peer" in the way it can influence perceptions about the prevalence and acceptance or disapproval of observed behaviors or beliefs. For example, traditional forms of media impacted youth substance use, with young people
being perceived as having more social approval for using alcohol and tobacco (Committee on Communications et al. 2006). Increasingly, social media operates as both a form of media and a peer, blending the two and
potentially magnifying the impact of two powerful influences.

Vulnerabilities That Heighten Risks

A common thread across the research that has explored the effects of social media on young people is that youth with certain "vulnerabilities" are more at risk for negative outcomes. Idelji-Tehrani et al. (2023) claimed that "children and young people who are particularly vulnerable online include those with family difficulties, disabilities, mental health difficulties, emotional/behavioral difficulties, and neurodevelopment disorders, as well as marginalised and disadvantaged groups" (p. 339). Indeed, it seems the youth most at risk online are also those most at risk offline (El Asam and Katz 2018). It also appears that interaction with the same media can affect two people very differently based on their individual susceptibilities and circumstances. The metaphor of the orchid and the dandelion has been used to illuminate the idea that some young people are more sensitive to environmental circumstances than others (Boyce and Ellis 2005)—that is, that a minority of young people are disproportionately negatively affected by adverse environmental forces but also thrive beautifully with positive inputs (orchids), whereas most are able to withstand a variety of environments in order to grow and thrive (dandelions). This paradigm of "differential susceptibility" proposes that one's responses to and selections of media are related to a confluence of dimensions that include "genetics, gender, temperament, personality, cognitions, values, attitudes, beliefs, motivations, and moods" (Piotrowski and Valkenburg 2015, p. 1779).

No one common definition of "vulnerable youth" has yet been established. Gaining more clarity on this issue will be important for identifying the points at which social media is helpful and harmful and how characteristics such as brain maturation, life experience, and the emergence of mental health conditions influence those points. The limited life experience of children and adolescents is often considered to be a vulnerability, particularly when they are presented with targeted advertising, illicit content, or complex social dynamics to navigate in social media spaces. Furthermore, the rapid changes that occur in the brain during adolescence create unique susceptibilities to influence that, in and of themselves, can be viewed as both vulnerabilities and opportunities for growth. The plasticity of the developing brain supports an incredible capacity for learning, and curiosity spurred by online exploration can lead to new interests, skills, and learning opportunities, which can be highly desirable outcomes within optimal circumstances (Ekman et al. 2022).

An example of where media can intersect with vulnerability is in the exposure to potentially traumatic events. Given a nonstop news cycle that covers violent and devastating events by the minute and billions of people uploading first-person videos to social media in real time, exposure to traumatic events via media is nearly impossible to avoid. Research supports the notion that some individuals will experience clinically significant secondary traumatic stress after viewing a traumatic event through media (Comstock and Platania 2017). In one study, nearly one-quarter of participants scored high on measures of PTSD despite having no prior history of trauma and only witnessing the events via social media. Effects were higher for those who reported more frequent viewing of the traumatic event (Muss 2017). We are all at risk for this indirect trauma every time we ingest news, and with media access so readily available, visual, and constant, this risk seems more heightened than ever.

For young people who are experiencing symptoms of mental health issues, engaging with social media offers a range of potential experiences that can include resources, advice, and support or can sometimes worsen feelings (Rideout et al. 2018). Experiences of mental ill health might introduce susceptibilities that need to be further explored and protected. Research indicates that young people with mental health issues turn to the internet for information, validation, and support and find both help and potentially harmful content online, including content that encourages or instructs self-harming and disordered eating (Stoilova et al. 2021). The internet is a common source of support for individuals who self-harm, and associations have been found between searches for self-harm/suicidal content and self-harm/suicidal behavior (Idelji-Tehrani et al. 2023). It seems that social media can be helpful or harmful depending on where a young person is on their spectrum of mental wellness or ill health and on their spectrum of accumulated vulnerability or resilience at the time they engage with it. Based on a series of consultations with young people, Livingstone et al. (2022) reported that

> platform algorithms are often "out of sync" with and insensitive to the young person's state of mind or ability to cope, leading to experiences of "triggering" (when particular online content proves upsetting because of prior mental health difficulties), unwanted re-exposure to such content, and setbacks in their mental health. Algorithms can act as a distorting mirror, magnifying problematic content and pushing young people with mental health vulnerabilities down a spiral of ever-more overwhelming, upsetting, or extreme content that they find hard to break away from. (p. 8)

Navigating triggering spaces and challenging content requires resilience and self-care, which many young people demonstrate in remarkable ways every day, but this remains an opportunity for clinicians, parents, and educators to better support youth.

Although research is still emerging, correlations have surfaced that warrant further exploration, particularly for youth with existing mental health risks. In addition to the developmental susceptibilities outlined earlier (see "Unique Considerations of the Adolescent Brain"), if the baseline mental health of the majority of the youth population indicates unprecedented levels of distress (60% of female students and 70% of LGBTQ+ students report "persistent feelings of sadness or hopelessness"; Centers for Disease Control and Prevention 2021), potential vulnerability is widespread; thus, policy and product decisions should default to prioritizing the health interests of youth. The World Health Organization (2021) estimates that one in seven 10- to 19-year-olds (14%) worldwide has a mental health condition. This adds up to an estimated 166 million adolescents globally (UNICEF 2021). With increasing access to social media and smartphones (nearly every teenager in the United States has access to a smartphone), this potentially vulnerable group includes millions of youth worldwide (Vogels et al. 2022). Until the potential mental health risks and gains associated with social media engagement are more fully understood, monitoring and proactively protecting the well-being of all should be a critical practice we adopt, with particular attention to young, vulnerable populations.

I first started using social media in middle school. None of the adults in my life had experience with these platforms at my age. They could not offer me advice about how to use these platforms while protecting my mental health and privacy. Since then, I have learned strategies to navigate social media while protecting my well-being through trial and error, conversations with my peers, and digital wellness campaigns like #GoodforMEdia.[*] Being able to name harmful behaviors and features that seemed like a "normal" part of the social media experience (e.g., social comparison, losing track of time while scrolling on social media)

---

[*] GoodforMEdia is a youth-driven, peer mentoring program that is designed to support young people's healthy engagement with technology and social media (visit www.goodformedia.org).

has been extremely empowering for me as I attempt to reshape my relationship with social media to benefit my
mental health.

—Sonia, age 17

Contagion

When considering the idea of vulnerabilities in some social media users, it
is important to factor in the contagion effect that media can inspire. Emotional contagion has been documented in digital environments, with exposure to the digitally expressed emotions of social media users affecting the
emotions and behaviors of others (Goldenberg and Gross 2020). Evidence
establishing a link between media depictions of suicide and increases in suicidal behavior has been established over many decades. Sensational media
coverage of suicides appears to induce copycat behavior in some individuals.
Suicide deaths reported by news media, particularly those of celebrities, has
been associated with an increase in suicides in the general population (Niederkrotenthaler et al. 2020). Niederkrotenthaler et al. (2020) found an 8%–
18% increase in suicide deaths in the 1–2 months following reporting on a
celebrity suicide and an increase of 18%–44% in the risk of suicide by the
same method when information about the suicide method was reported.

These data highlight the substantial evidence base that spurred the World
Health Organization and suicide prevention and journalism communities to
establish journalistic reporting guidelines for suicide in an effort to save lives
(World Health Organization and International Association for Suicide Prevention 2017). Eating disorder associations worldwide have followed suit,
establishing media guidelines to minimize the contagion that media content
can trigger in those struggling with or vulnerable to disordered eating behaviors (Mindframe 2021). These guidelines share common recommendations that include minimizing descriptive details about methods, carefully
selecting photos and language, and promoting crisis lines and help-seeking.

Although these guidelines were originally established when traditional
media dominated, the risks within a social media context appear higher, possibly more pronounced, and less manageable. As indicated earlier (see "Vulnerabilities That Heighten Risks"), some self-harming and suicidal youth
seek social support by engaging in social media and, in doing so, can be exposed to content and videos that promote and encourage self-injurious behavior. For these vulnerable adolescents, greater time spent on social media

platforms is linked with higher psychological distress and increased suicidal ideation (Memon et al. 2018). Social media platforms are frequently used for self-harm, eating disorder, and suicide-related content, representing a significant public health risk, particularly if one considers the number of social media users who are uniquely susceptible to its exposure (Carlyle et al. 2018). For example, in a given year, suicidal thoughts are common among about 4% of the U.S. population (Niederkrotenthaler et al. 2020), with a notable 22% of high school students having seriously considered suicide in the past year (Centers for Disease Control and Prevention 2021), suggesting that many people are vulnerable to the media's contagion effect. The mental health community is long overdue in adapting media guidelines for suicide contagion into a social media context. To empower industry and social media users to adopt best practices and avoid a piecemeal approach, it would be beneficial to adopt a holistic set of guidelines that account for a multitude of areas in which a contagion effect has been observed or appears likely, including disordered eating, self-harm, and online challenges.

Beyond What's on the Screen

Although the effects of social media content on youth mental health continue to be at the foreground of societal debates, the cultural norms that have been adopted for social media use over the past two decades are worthy of more consideration. Take a moment to consider some of the social norms that the age of social media has ushered in:

- Continuously documenting and posting photos of daily activities via selfies.
- Measuring status by the numbers of follows, likes, views, and shares for both everyday users and influencers who are compensated according to that "status."
- Consuming daily news and posts that have been determined by opaque algorithmic tailoring and filtering.
- Expecting immediate feedback to texts and social media posts.
- Exposing ourselves to and communicating with thousands of strangers and large extended networks of people on a daily basis.
- Some parents giving cellular phones to young people at young ages as a rite of passage, in some cases allowing unfettered access, versus a minority of parents restricting or denying youth cell phone access, either of which brings new challenges to parenting (and youth).

- Self-publishing plus algorithmic "virality" obscuring previously held barometers of truth and neutral facts, placing unprecedented demands on both media and media literacy education.
- Engaging with social media in the most popular and most-used platforms at the cost of losing privacy and control of personal data, with no option to withhold that data.

I tend to feel apologetic if I notice I didn't respond very quickly to a message, as do my friends. Furthermore, I also see lots of youth online who will apologize for not responding "fast enough." This does indeed create a pressured digital life and raises already high expectations. We've succumbed to society's pressured digital life.

—Violet, age 13

The ubiquitous use of smartphones and social media has served up a one-two punch of social transformation that we have not fully considered as it relates to youth well-being. It is possible that the behaviors and expectations associated with media use are as influential and challenging as the content consumed. For instance, the "quantification of social acceptance," calculated through measures such as follower counts, likes, and shares, can negatively impact self-perceptions and the mental health of young people (Idelji-Tehrani et al. 2023). In one particular analysis of Instagram (Cipolletta et al. 2020), increases in social isolation and self-esteem were associated with receiving or not receiving likes, suggesting that the feedback youth receive on posts impacts their self-perception more than use of the platform itself. This fact supports the growing body of evidence that social media participation can have both beneficial and harmful effects on youth depending on the number of interactions they have and the reactions they experience, as well as the individual characteristics and contexts of those interactions.

Another influential cultural norm to consider is how the immediacy of messaging through text and chat features has set up an expectation that response times should be immediate or very short. This norm creates a pressure and relationship expectation that is completely independent of the content of the message itself. That expectation, in turn, feeds feelings of overwhelm and pressure for young people to constantly keep up with their incoming and outgoing messaging and works against healthy habits, such as disconnecting for periods of time during the day or evening or choosing to engage with deliberate intention rather than reflexively in response to persistent notifications. If constantly connected to their peers and barraged with media messages, will young people be able to define their individuality and resist the influences of "media-centered and media-facilitated peer culture" (Lim 2013)? Could a shift in expectations create a sense of relief and balance for the next generation? We need to settle on healthy cultural norms for both the content with which we interact and the shape and frequency with which those interactions occur. According to participatory research with young people in Australia, online safety education that meets the needs of young people would cover a wide-ranging set of skill development categories: communicating effectively; building respectful relationships; establishing, maintaining, and respecting boundaries; and cultivating resilience and critical thinking (Marsden et al. 2022).

> Whether it be my email inbox, texts, or Instagram DMs [direct messages], I've always experienced an overwhelming sense of discomfort and anxiety opening and responding to virtual communication. I find myself constantly apologizing for getting back to people late or missing a message, and it makes me feel inferior compared to my friends and coworkers. It seems like everyone around me has mastered this essential skill; meanwhile, I have yet to make any meaningful progress with my apprehension. Unfortunately, this unspoken expectation translates to tension and guilt in my face-to-face interactions. I don't want anyone to feel that they are the reason I'm not responding. I promise—it's not you, it's me!
>
> —*Kyra, age 21*

Looking Ahead

The influence that omnipresent media has in the lives of children and young adults raises many questions about the extent to which the potential effects of media should be mediated to maximize benefits and minimize harms. As discussed, the heightened sensitivity of the adolescent brain is justification for regarding young people as a vulnerable group that needs safer, more supportive, and developmentally scaffolded social media experiences. Barsotti and Koçer (2022) proposed that algorithmic decision-making should consider the most vulnerable, aiming to increase the benefit for less advantaged groups, and that doing so is possible in a way that serves all participants.

This is echoed in the Child Online Safety Toolkit, a consolidation of four international sets of guidelines and agreements, including the United Nations Committee on the Rights of the Child's general comment 25, which names "identifying risk and mitigating harm" as one of its five core principles. It states that

> children around the world will face many of the same risks, but some are more vulnerable to harm due to their location, gender, age, family circumstances, socioeconomic status, and availability of digital technology. Identifying risks and mitigating them by design is a key principle of child online safety. (5Rights Foundation 2022)

Although its unintended impacts are still coming into focus, the dominant influence of media in the lives of young people is unmistakable. There are well-known instances of aligning media practices, policies, and content with public health priorities, such as limiting exposure to commercial advertising or content showing alcohol, drugs, and sexual content (Committee on Communications et al. 2006). The social media ecosystem is not yet adequately scaffolded to protect and support young people, a uniquely vulnerable population due to characteristics of the adolescent brain, the power of peer influence, and other developmental attributes. On this important matter, the public health and child rights perspectives align and must work with industry, government leaders, and youth themselves to inspire improvements in policy and product design.

References

Anderson CA, Berkowitz L, Donnerstein E, et al: The influence of media violence on youth. Psychol Sci Public Interest 4(3):81–110, 2003 26151870

Barsotti F, Koçer RG: MinMax fairness: from Rawlsian theory of justice to solution for algorithmic bias. AI Soc, November 2022

Becker AE: Television, disordered eating, and young women in Fiji: negotiating body image and identity during rapid social change. Cult Med Psychiatry 28(4):533–559, 2004 15847053

Becker AE, Fay KE, Agnew-Blais J, et al: Social network media exposure and adolescent eating pathology in Fiji. Br J Psychiatry 198(1):43–50, 2011 21200076

Boyce WT, Ellis BJ: Biological sensitivity to context: I. An evolutionary-developmental theory of the origins and functions of stress reactivity. Dev Psychopathol 17(2):271–301, 2005 16761546

Bryant J, Oliver MB (eds): Media Effects, 3rd Edition. New York, Routledge, 2008

Carlyle KE, Guidry JPD, Williams K, et al: Suicide conversations on Instagram: contagion or caring? J Commun Healthc 11(1):12–18, 2018

Centers for Disease Control and Prevention: Youth Risk Behavior Survey Data Summary and Trends Report 2011–2021. Atlanta, GA, Centers for Disease Control and Prevention, 2021. Available at: https://www.cdc.gov/healthyyouth/data/yrbs/pdf/YRBS_Data-Summary-Trends_Report2023_508.pdf. Accessed November 20, 2023.

Cipolletta S, Malighetti C, Cenedese C, et al: How can adolescents benefit from the use of social networks? The iGeneration on Instagram. Int J Environ Res Public Health 17(19):6952, 2020 32977532

Committee on Communications, American Academy of Pediatrics, Strasburger VC: Children, adolescents, and advertising. Pediatrics 118(6):2563–2569, 2006 17142547

Comstock C, Platania J: The role of media-induced secondary traumatic stress on perceptions of distress. American International Journal of Social Science 16(1):1–10, 2017

Datareportal: Digital Around the World. Singapore, Kepios, 2023. Available at: https://datareportal.com/global-digital-overview. Accessed March 3, 2023.

Ekman R, Fletcher A, Giota J, et al: A flourishing brain in the 21st century: a scoping review of the impact of developing good habits for mind, brain, well-being, and learning. Mind Brain Educ 16(1):13–23, 2022

El Asam A, Katz A: Vulnerable young people and their experience of online risks. Hum Comput Interact 33(4):281–304, 2018

Elmore KC, Scull TM, Kupersmidt JB: Media as a "super peer": how adolescents interpret media messages predicts their perception of alcohol and tobacco use norms. J Youth Adolesc 46(2):376–387, 2017 27837371

Fardouly J, Pinkus RT, Vartanian LR: The impact of appearance comparisons made through social media, traditional media, and in person in women's everyday lives. Body Image 20(March):31–39, 2017 27907812

5Rights Foundation: Child Online Safety Toolkit. London, 5Rights Foundation, 2022. Available at: https://childonlinesafetytoolkit.org/about. Accessed November 20, 2023.

Giordano AL, Schmit MK, Clement K, et al: Pornography use and sexting trends among American adolescents: data to inform school counseling programming and practice. Professional School Counseling 26(1):1–11, 2022

Goldenberg A, Gross JJ: Digital emotion contagion. Trends Cogn Sci 24(4):316–328, 2020 32160568

Goodyear VA, Armour KM: Young people's health-related learning through social media: what do teachers need to know? Teach Teach Educ 102(June):103340, 2021 34083866

Grubbs JB, Kraus SW: Pornography use and psychological science: a call for consideration. Curr Dir Psychol Sci 30(1):68–75, 2021

Idelji-Tehrani S, Dubicka B, Graham R: The clinical implications of digital technology. Clin Child Psychol Psychiatry 28(1):338–353, 2023 36525979

Ito M, Martin C, Pfister RC, et al: Affinity Online: How Connection and Shared Interest Fuel Learning, Vol 2. New York, NYU Press, 2018

Lim S: Media and peer culture: young people sharing norms and collective identities with and through media, in The Routledge Handbook of Children, Adolescents, and Media. Edited by Lemish D. New York, Routledge, 2013, pp 322–328

Livingstone S, Stoilova M, Stänicke LI, et al: Young People Experiencing Internet-Related Mental Health Difficulties: The Benefits and Risks of Digital Skills: An

Empirical Study. KU Leuven, ySKILLS, 2022. Available at: https:// www.hf.uio.no/imk/english/research/center/children-media/publications/ reports/yskills/d6.1---young-people-experiencing-internet-related-mental-health-difficulties.pdf. Accessed November 20, 2023.

Lombana-Bermudez A, Cortesi S, Fieseler C, et al: Youth and the Digital Economy: Exploring Youth Practices, Motivations, Skills, Pathways, and Value Creation. Cambridge, MA, Youth and Media, Berkman Klein Center for Internet and Society, 2020. Available at: https://dash.harvard.edu/handle/1/42669835. Accessed November 20, 2023.

Marino C, Gini G, Angelini F, et al: Social norms and e-motions in problematic social media use among adolescents. Addict Behav Rep 11(June):100250, 2020 32467839

Marsden L, Moody L, Nguyen B, et al: Reimagining Online Safety Education Through the Eyes of Young People: Co-Design Workshops With Young People to Inform Digital Learning Experiences. Penrith, Australia, Western Sydney University, 2022. Available at: https://researchdirect.westernsydney.edu.au/ islandora/object/uws:68382. Accessed November 20, 2023.

Memon AM, Sharma SG, Mohite SS, et al: The role of online social networking on deliberate self-harm and suicidality in adolescents: a systematized review of literature. Indian J Psychiatry 60(4):384–392, 2018 30581202

Mindframe: Guidelines on Reporting and Portrayal of Eating Disorders: A Mindframe Resource for Communicators. Newcastle, New South Wales, Australia, Everymind, 2021. Available at: https://www.nedc.com.au/assets/NEDC-Resources/ Collaborative-Resources/NEDC-Mindframe-Reporting-Guidelines.pdf. Accessed November 20, 2023.

Muss D: The international association for rewind trauma therapy. J Depress Anxiety 06(3 Suppl), 2017

Niederkrotenthaler T, Braun M, Pirkis J, et al: Association between suicide reporting in the media and suicide: systematic review and meta-analysis. BMJ 368(March):m575, 2020 32188637

Orben A: Teenagers, screens and social media: a narrative review of reviews and key studies. Soc Psychiatry Psychiatr Epidemiol 55(4):407–414, 2020 31925481

Paus-Hasebrink I, Kulterer J, Sinner P: Social Inequality, Childhood, and the Media: A Longitudinal Study of the Mediatization of Socialisation. Transforming Communications—Studies in Cross-Media Research. Cham, Switzerland, Springer International, 2019

Perkins HW, Craig DW, Perkins JM: Using social norms to reduce bullying: a research intervention among adolescents in five middle schools. Group Process Intergroup Relat 14(5):703–722, 2011

Piotrowski JT, Valkenburg PM: Finding orchids in a field of dandelions: understanding children's differential susceptibility to media effects. Am Behav Sci 59(14):1776–1789, 2015

Przybylski AK, Weinstein N: Violent video game engagement is not associated with adolescents' aggressive behaviour: evidence from a registered report. R Soc Open Sci 6(2):171474, 2019 30891250

Radesky J, Chassiakos YLR, Ameenuddin N, et al: Digital advertising to children. Pediatrics 146(1):e20201681, 2020 32571990

Reidy M: 78% of influencers admit to suffering burnout. AWIN, August 22, 2022. Available at: https://www.awin.com/us/news-and-events/industry-news/creator-burnout-survey. Accessed November 20, 2023.

Rideout V, Fox S, Well Being Trust: Digital health practices, social media use, and mental well-being among teens and young adults in the U.S. Well Being Trust, July 31, 2018. Available at: https://wellbeingtrust.org/bewell/digital-health-practices-social-media-use-and-mental-well-being-among-teens-and-young-adults-in-the-u-s. Accessed November 20, 2023.

Robb MB, Mann S: 2022: Teens and Pornography. San Francisco, CA, Common Sense Media, 2023

Stoilova M, Edwards C, Kostyrka-Allchorne K, et al: Adolescents' Mental Health Vulnerabilities and the Experience and Impact of Digital Technologies: A Multimethod Pilot Study. London, London School of Economics and Political Science, 2021

Telzer EH, Dai J, Capella JJ, et al: Challenging stereotypes of teens: reframing adolescence as window of opportunity. Am Psychol 77(9):1067–1081, 2022 36595405

Thurman N, Obster F: The regulation of internet pornography: what a survey of under-18s tells us about the necessity for and potential efficacy of emerging legislative approaches. Policy Internet 13(3):415–432, 2021

Tibber MS, Silver E: A trans-diagnostic cognitive behavioural conceptualisation of the positive and negative roles of social media use in adolescents' mental health and wellbeing. Cogn Behav Therap 15:e7, 2022

Tudge JRH, Winterhoff PA: Vygotsky, Piaget, and Bandura: perspectives on the relations between the social world and cognitive development. Hum Dev 36(2):61–81, 1993

UNICEF: Ensuring mental health and well-being in an adolescent's formative years can foster a better transition from childhood to adulthood. Mental Health, updated October 2021. Available at: https://data.unicef.org/topic/child-health/mental-health/#_edn1. Accessed November 20, 2023.

Valkenburg PM, Meier A, Beyens I: Social media use and its impact on adolescent mental health: an umbrella review of the evidence. Curr Opin Psychol 44(April):58–68, 2022 34563980

Vogels EA, Gelles-Watnick R, Massarat N: Teens, social media and technology: acknowledgments. Pew Research Center, August 10, 2022. Available at: https://www.pewresearch.org/internet/2022/08/10/teens-and-tech-acknowledgments. Accessed November 17, 2023.

Wartella E, Beaudoin-Ryan L, Blackwell CK, et al: What kind of adults will our children become? The impact of growing up in a media-saturated world. J Child Media 10(1):13–20, 2016

Weinstein E, James C: Behind Their Screens: What Teens Are Facing (and Adults Are Missing). Cambridge, MA, MIT Press, 2022

World Health Organization: Adolescent Mental Health. Geneva, World Health Organization, November 17, 2021. Available at: https://www.who.int/news-room/fact-sheets/detail/adolescent-mental-health. Accessed November 20, 2023.

World Health Organization, International Association for Suicide Prevention: Preventing Suicide: A Resource for Media Professionals, 2017 Update. Geneva,

World Health Organization, 2017. Available at: https://apps.who.int/iris/handle/10665/258814. Accessed November 20, 2023.

Young HP: The evolution of social norms. Annu Rev Econ 7(1):359–387, 2015

2

Sexuality and Media

Exploration and Exploitation

Chelly Maes, Ph.D.
Faith Arimoro, M.P.H.
Linda Charmaraman, Ph.D.

Next to the support of peers and parents, digital media is an important tool with the potential to facilitate the challenging process of youth's sexual development. In this chapter, we shed light on the impressive line of research exploring the impact of youth's sexual digital media activities (i.e., relationship dynamics online, [non-]consensual sexting, and pornography use). Moreover, we pay attention to the internet's role for LGBTQ+ youth.

Some research reported in this chapter was supported by the Eunice Kennedy Shriver National Institute of Child Health and Human Development of the National Institutes of Health under award number 1R15HD094281-01 to the third author (L.C.). The content is solely the responsibility of the authors and does not necessarily represent the official views of the National Institutes of Health. Also, some research reported here was supported by the Bijzonder Onderzoeksfonds KU Leuven (grant number C14/18/017), and some of the work of putting together this chapter was funded through a FOCUS Medical Student Fellowship in Women's Health, supported by the Bertha Dagan Berman Award at the University of Pennsylvania.

Relationship Dynamics in Online Spaces

Digital media plays a key role in initiating and maintaining relationships among adolescents. For many youth, online dating facilitates meeting new partners and is especially helpful for socially reserved adolescents who may be more likely to initiate romantic relationships online (Tienda et al. 2022). Social media is often a key tool in helping potential partners determine compatibility; various sites allow someone to identify a potential partner's social network, hobbies, and self-presentation—something referred to by some as "doing your homework" (Howard et al. 2019).

Once relationships are initiated, phone calls, text messages, and online chats are integral ways adolescents maintain them and can help promote relationship satisfaction. A survey of 1,960 dating youth in grades 7–12 found that time spent interacting via a computer or cellular phone predicted positive relationship quality with a romantic partner (Mosley and Lancaster 2019). Particularly in the early days of a relationship, instant messaging can reduce feelings of uncertainty and insecurity (Sánchez-Jiménez et al. 2020).

On the other hand, digital media can be harmful to developing relationships in several ways. One example is that online platforms can enable deception: hiding one's relationship status online can facilitate infidelity. In addition, some scholars argue that dating applications (apps) weaken interpersonal ties and limit someone's ability to interact with others offline (Duguay 2017).

> [M]illennials don't really communicate well with people outside of our phone. So, it's just easier. If I was gonna meet a guy, this [Tinder] would be the way to do it.
>
> —*Talia, age 20* (Christensen 2021)

Furthermore, some teens describe social media as a convenient platform for fueling interpersonal conflict, albeit not necessarily the precipitating factor.

> [A] guy is dating a girl, but there's a picture of him hugging a girl at a party or something, then that can create problems... and I feel like people use the internet to just create drama that doesn't need to be there.
>
> —*anonymous, age 15* (Howard et al. 2019)

Additionally, the ease of accessibility for digital platforms creates some degree of pressure to be constantly connected to them (Howard et al. 2019). One systematic review of studies investigating the relationship between social media use and adolescent mental health found that increased time spent on social media may be associated with increased rates of depression, anxiety, and psychological distress (Keles et al. 2020). Moreover, the need to constantly monitor and be monitored may make adolescents more susceptible to harmful relationship dynamics to the point of abuse. Monitoring and control are the most prevalent forms of technology-facilitated abuse, with females more likely to use controlling behaviors in their dating relationships. Examples of monitoring behaviors include pressuring a partner to respond quickly to a text or monitoring a partner's activities and friendships (Ellyson et al. 2021).

Many studies have demonstrated that individuals who are perpetrators of technology-facilitated abuse are often also victims of this abuse (Brown et al. 2021; Ellyson et al. 2021). For instance, females who use certain forms of abuse such as monitoring and control can also experience other forms of abuse, such as sexual coercion. Young females are more likely to report experiencing insults or pressure to have sex or send sexual photos while in a relationship (Reed et al. 2020). Unfortunately, this form of abuse of females is so prevalent in some online spaces that it is considered to be part of the culture. One qualitative study examining stories of abuse noted that a number of females had experienced verbal abuse, unwanted graphic pictures, and crude sexual solicitations (Thompson 2018). Threats are less common than other forms of technology-facilitated abuse but can be particularly disruptive to an individual's well-being when they do occur. Examples include one partner threatening suicide or threatening physical violence toward the other partner's family to extort sexual favors. Of the four categories of technology-facilitated abuse (including humiliation, monitoring and control, sexual coercion, and threats) examined in one study, threats were determined to cause the most amount of distress and fear for both males and females (Brown et al. 2021).

Technology-facilitated abuse can have an impact not only on relationship quality but also on individual health. Brown et al. (2021) found that victims of technology-facilitated abuse reported lower scores on quality-of-life measures, lower self-esteem, and heightened emotional distress. Adolescents are particularly vulnerable to technology-facilitated abuse because many of them have limited relationship experience and limited knowledge of what constitutes healthy relationship behaviors (Brown et al. 2021). For many youth, adolescence marks a time when some relationships move from friendship to casual dating to committed relationships. This transition can be difficult and may contribute to feelings of jealousy, insecurity, and frustration. Complicating things, partners may perceive their level of investment in a relationship as being unequal. This emotionally fragile backdrop can be fertile ground for falling prey to technology-facilitated abuse (Baker and Carreño 2016). In addition, several studies have demonstrated a correlation between cyber-abuse and offline abuse (Cava et al. 2020; Erevik et al. 2020).

Finally, dating apps can reproduce systems of power imbalance. For instance, one study of college students' experiences with the dating app Tinder showed that racial minority students often experienced explicit racial and sexual discrimination on the app (Christensen 2021).

> The "wanna fuck?" thing is usually from White guys, and I'm not sure—maybe they do that to all women, but it feels like they see me as some kind of Jezebel, like I'm easy to sleep with.
> —*Aleia, age 24* (Christensen 2021)

Consensual Sexting and Nonconsensual Image-Sharing

The emergence of digital media brought sexting into young people's sexual experiences. In the literature, *sexting* is generally described as "the online sending of self-made sexually explicit messages, images, and videos" (Van Ouytsel et al. 2019). Yet recent voices have suggested that sexting cannot be considered a single behavior; rather, distinctions should be made between different sexting types according to variations in sexual explicitness (Maes and Vandenbosch 2022b). Youth may prefer to experiment with less explicit forms of sexting first (e.g., textual) before engaging in more explicit types (e.g., nude photos or depiction of sexual acts via video). Regardless of the specific type, research shows that, worldwide, a sizable minority of adolescents and youth engage in this online sexual behavior. Particularly, 14.8% of adolescents send sexts and 27.4% receive sexts (Madigan et al. 2018), while 38.3% of young adults send sexts and 41.5% receive sexts (Mori et al. 2020).

When discussing young people's sexting, it is important to make a distinction between consensual and nonconsensual sexting (Mori et al. 2020). *Consensual sexting* takes place between two sexual/romantic partners who both consent to engage in this behavior. Youth usually engage in consensual sexting to address developmental needs (e.g., sexual identity exploration) and to initiate or to maintain a relationship (Cooper et al. 2016; Maes and Vandenbosch 2022b). Research into youth's sexuality-related outcomes of consensual sexting is still relatively scarce, but emerging. Studies point to links between youth's consensual sexting and a more developed self-concept (i.e., understanding one's sexual self) (Marengo et al. 2019), greater sexual satisfaction (Galovan et al. 2018), and a higher feeling of sexual attraction, passion, and arousal toward one's partner (Van Ouytsel et al. 2019). Furthermore, sexting seems to be related to a higher frequency of sexual activities (MacDonald et al. 2018), having multiple sexual partners (e.g., Romo et al. 2017), and engaging in unsafe sexual behaviors (no contraceptive use) (Rice et al. 2018). Contrary to public concerns about adolescent sexting, at least one study has shown that 92% of non-pressured sexting was not associated with any negative consequences (Englander 2012).

Nonconsensual sexting occurs when someone is coerced into sexting under threats or pressure by a partner or someone they do not know (Wolak et al. 2018). Recent reports indicate that 7.2% of adolescents have been victims of nonconsensual sexting (Finkelhor et al. 2022). Females, adult females in particular, experience (implicit) pressure to send sexually explicit pictures or videos of themselves because sexual double standards suggest they must be sexually attractive to maintain or initiate a relationship (Lippman and Campbell 2014). Thus, they are more inclined to send sexts to attract a partner. Yet, concurrently, moral responsibility is attributed more to females for sending such a picture (Ringrose et al. 2013), and young females are more likely to be slut-shamed when a nude photograph is leaked (Weinstein and James 2022). Thus, online activities of young females seem to be subjected to sexist norms (Lippman and Campbell 2014). Young males experience peer pressure to engage in sexting because obtaining sexts from young females can increase a male's popularity (Ringrose et al. 2013). Furthermore, research suggests that gender and sexual minority youth are at higher risk of becoming victims of abusive sexting practices (e.g., pressured sexting) (Van Ouytsel et al. 2020). Although scarce, some literature has shown that pressured sexting was related to more depressive symptoms and self-harm, whereas consensual sexting was not related to such outcomes (Wachs et al. 2021). Research investigating sexuality-related outcomes of pressured sexting is still in its infancy.

When, like, girls take a picture of their breasts and stuff, that is why most boys call them slags and stuff because they...have

> no respect for themselves and they know that obviously the
> boy is going to show their close friends.
>   —*Danvir, age 15* (Ringrose et al. 2013)

With sexting comes the risk of one's sexts being forwarded to audiences other than the intended recipient without the sender's consent (Walker and Sleath 2017). Recent reports indicate that 8.4% of adolescents (Madigan et al. 2018) and 7.6% of young adults (Mori et al. 2020) have been the victim of nonconsensual forwarding of their sexts. Furthermore, 12% of adolescents (Madigan et al. 2018) and 23% of young adults (Garcia et al. 2016) have admitted to having forwarded sexts without receiving consent from the creator. Victim-blaming beliefs (e.g., overestimating the victim's own responsibility for their sexts being forwarded) appear to be an important contributor to the nonconsensual forwarding of sexts among youth (Maes et al. 2023a), as well as several personality factors, including narcissism and Machiavellianism (Morelli et al. 2016), which are part of the dark triad of personality. Research to date has mainly attended to the well-being-related risks of having one's sext forwarded without their consent and points to close links with poor mental well-being, suicidality indicators, and interpersonal violence (e.g., Pampati et al. 2020). As for sexuality-related outcomes, research is still lacking.

A recent study by Finkelhor et al. (2022) shed light on a variety of activities surrounding sexual image misuse among youth (e.g., nonconsensual sharing, taking, and threatened sharing of sexting messages). Sexual image misuse was associated with heightened negative emotions (e.g., feeling angry, afraid, sad) and mainly appeared to be perpetrated by peers. The impact of peer sexual image misuse on youth was equally as detrimental as sexual image misuse by adult offenders.

Pornography Use

Youth consider pornographic online content an appealing source of sexual material because it is accessible and can be used anonymously (Wright 2014). *Pornography* can generally be described as "professionally produced or user-generated pictures or videos intended to sexually arouse the viewer" (Peter and Valkenburg 2011, pp. 1015–1016). Recent reports show the relatively high prevalence of pornography use among both adolescents (in the United States, 77% of young males and 33% of young females watch pornography; similar rates have been found in Europe; Hardy et al. 2019; Maes and Vandenbosch 2022a) and young adults (94.1% of males, 86.9% of females in the United States; Herbenick et al. 2020). A recent survey of 1,300 adolescents found that nearly one-third (31%) had viewed pornography while at school and that 15% had consumed pornography before the age of 11 (Robb and Mann 2023). Youth primarily turn to pornography to 1) gratify themselves sexually, 2) gratify their growing sexual curiosity and explore their sexual selves, 3) gain information regarding sexual activities in general, and 4) regulate their emotions (e.g., stress, boredom, loneliness) (Bőthe et al. 2020).

Research has mainly been driven by concerns regarding the socializing potential of pornography. Such concerns are rooted in the biased and unrealistic content embedded in pornography. Particularly, content analytical work describes how pornography frequently depicts solely sexual satisfaction (e.g., in casual sex situations), ignoring the emotional and physical complexities tied to sexual interactions. Scholars have also warned of pornographic content's neglect of safe sexual practices (e.g., use of contraceptives) and reinforcement of sexual gender stereotypes (e.g., Fritz and Paul 2017). In particular, research has shown that, in online pornographic content, the women are more sexually submissive than the men, are sexually objectified (Fritz and Paul 2017), and are the target of verbal and physical aggression (Bridges et al. 2010).

> M1: It is kind of weird…
> M2: Girls are inferior.
> M3: It doesn't have to be like that, but it is often that way….
> Well, the guy says to the girl: "Do that and that!" Most of the times, the girl does everything for the guy!
> *—Male focus group, ages 17–20*
> (Lofgren-Mårtenson and Månsson 2010)

Building on this content analytical work, a great body of cross-sectional and experimental work and some longitudinal research have explored how pornography use can be detrimental for youth's sexual attitudes and behaviors. Research has consistently shown how young people's use of pornography negatively affects the degree to which they are satisfied with their own sexual lives (Wright et al. 2017). These links appear to be the strongest among youth with little to no sexual experience and are often only found among male participants (Wright et al. 2017). Furthermore, more frequent pornography viewing can be related to higher uncertainties surrounding one's sexual beliefs and attitudes (Peter and Valkenburg 2016). This link often occurs via experiences of involvement with pornographic content (Peter and Valkenburg 2010), and young females appear to be more often affected than young males (van Oosten 2016). Other attitudinal outcomes of youth's pornography use include increases in sexually permissive attitudes (i.e., toward sex with casual partners; e.g., Peter and Valkenburg 2016), gender stereotypical and sexist beliefs (e.g., Robb and Mann 2023), and objectifying beliefs (especially toward females; e.g., Maes et al. 2019). The latter beliefs even explain the relationships between pornography use and the acceptance of rape myths (Maes et al. 2019). As for behavioral outcomes, literature shows that the more youth watch pornography, the earlier their sexual initiation and the higher their likelihood of having (casual) sexual intercourse with multiple sexual partners (e.g., Donevan and Mattebo 2017). Some studies further point to associations with sexual aggression (pressuring another person into having sex despite nonconsent) (Wright et al. 2021).

More recent and emerging work seeks to examine the *positive* impact of young people's pornography use, based on the reasoning that the exclusive focus on negative outcomes needs to be balanced. For instance, a study by Klein et al. (2020) demonstrated the positive potential of young females' pornography consumption. Specifically, it appears that the more young females watch pornographic content online, the higher their feelings of sexual agency. Relatedly, recent research points to the necessity of distinguishing among different pornographic genres, based on the reasoning that some genres are more biased and violent than others (e.g., paraphilic pornography) and therefore may be related to different outcomes. In this view, Maes et al. (2023b) demonstrated that viewing mainstream pornography, and not paraphilic pornography, can be related to a higher sexual arousability over time (i.e., the degree to which one can feel sexual excitation in any given situation, apart from using pornography). More work is necessary, however, to unravel the positive potential of pornography, especially by distinguishing different pornographic genres.

LGBTQ+ Youth's Experiences in the Online Sphere

Given the history of LGBTQ+ youth being more vulnerable to cybervictimization and the risks of coming out or the fear of losing access to their smartphones or social media (Cooper and Blumenfeld 2012), studies have also found that, compared with their heteronormative counterparts, LGBTQ+ youth are more private, prefer smaller online networks, are less likely to engage and connect, and are less likely to be online friends with their family members and peers (Charmaraman et al. 2022). The content they consume is also of concern—sexual minority youth are more likely to report seeing online content related to self-harm and are also more likely to attempt self-harm (Charmaraman et al. 2021).

Digital media may also be a source of resilience for members of sexual and gender minority groups. Digital media has provided LGBTQ+ users with spaces to co-construct identities with like-minded others and to share content with one another. Prior research has found that LGBTQ+ adolescents as young as 13, on average, spend more time online than their heterosexual, cisgender counterparts (Palmer et al. 2013). A study of 1,033 youth ages 10–16 in which 24.3% identified as LGBTQ+ showed that, compared with their heteronormative peers, LGBTQ+ youth were significantly more likely to use social media and online communities to feel less lonely (Charmaraman et al. 2021). During the social distancing period of the coronavirus disease 2019 (COVID-19) pandemic, this reliance on social media only grew stronger. Whereas nearly one-third (29%) of LGBTQ+ youth reported using social media to make them feel less alone during pre-pandemic times (fall 2019), 59% reported the same during pandemic times (summer 2022). Queer youth may feel excluded in traditional media and thus be more motivated to seek community online (Belfort 2022). One study of 130 transgender and gender-diverse adolescents found that almost 80% had used a website or app to seek a partner (Ma et al. 2022). In contrast to offline interactions, online platforms enable these young people to more easily maintain autonomy in disclosing their sexual orientation or gender identity and disengage from uncomfortable interactions (Ma et al. 2022).

Prior research has revealed that LGBTQ+ youth tend to gravitate toward particular sites such as Tumblr, which, due to its features, enables them to connect with others in the LGBTQ+ community with minimal threat of exposing their identities and with the emphasis on content *sharing* over content *creation* (Cavalcante 2019). In one of our interview studies, a participant remarked laughingly that Tumblr is "probably the gayest site ever that's not actually for gay people."

Conclusion

Uses of online media have consistently been shown to shape youth's sexual self-development, romantic relationships, sexual attitudes, and sexual behaviors. Canvassing the literature has surfaced several suggestions that can be made for future research. First, we encourage clinicians and researchers to pay more attention to the beneficial implications of digital media uses for youth's sexuality. Prior research has predominantly focused on the negative outcomes of online media use in the realm of youth's sexuality. Yet a small body of emerging research also points to the positive potential of online media, including the use of digital spaces to shape one's sexual identity. Thus, there is a substantial need to listen to youth's voices urging parents and concerned adults to recognize youth's sexual agency with regard to consensual sexting and online sexuality exploration. Clinicians and youth development workers who present an open-minded, judgment-free, and curious attitude and who make room for patients to explore positive sexual outcomes (e.g., sexual agency) can increase opportunities to expand our existing knowledge of youth's experiences with online media. Second and relatedly, the investigation of underlying processes explaining sexuality-related effects of online media uses and its conditional boundaries should be considered crucial. By paying attention to 1) how and 2) under which conditions sexuality-related effects of online media are formed, we can reach a more comprehensive understanding of the digital world as far as sex and sexuality are concerned. Furthermore, when it comes to the socializing potential of youth's pornography use, only a few empirical studies have taken a content-specific approach (e.g., Maes et al. 2023b). This leaves little room for providing nuance according to the content youth consume. We therefore recommend that pornography research pay attention to the unique outcomes tied to the consumption of specific pornography genres (e.g., paraphilic, mainstream pornography).

We also encourage future research to adopt longitudinal and daily-diary research designs when exploring the impact of online sexual media uses. Such designs can provide in-depth insights regarding, respectively, the durable relationships between and daily fluctuations in youth's online media uses and sexuality-related attitudes and behaviors. Moreover, they can shed additional light on the possible bidirectional nature of links between youth's online media uses and sexuality-related outcomes.

References

Baker C, Carreño PK: Understanding the role of technology in adolescent dating and dating violence. J Child Fam Stud 25(1):308–320, 2016

Belfort EL: 4.2 Social media as the contemporary medium for exploration of adolescent "self" (identity) and "other" (sexuality). J Am Acad Child Adolesc Psychiatry 61(10 Suppl):S130, 2022

Bőthe B, Tóth-Király I, Potenza MN, et al: High-frequency pornography use may not always be problematic. J Sex Med 17(4):793–811, 2020 32033863

Bridges AJ, Wosnitzer R, Scharrer E, et al: Aggression and sexual behavior in best-selling pornography videos: a content analysis update. Violence Against Women 16(10):1065–1085, 2010 20980228

Brown C, Sanci L, Hegarty K: Technology-facilitated abuse in relationships: victim-isation patterns and impact in young people. Comput Human Behav 124:11, 2021

Cava M-J, Martínez-Ferrer B, Buelga S, et al: Sexist attitudes, romantic myths, and offline dating violence as predictors of cyber dating violence perpetration in ad-olescents. Comput Human Behav 111:11, 2020

Cavalcante A: Tumbling into queer utopias and vortexes: experiences of LGBTQ so-cial media users on Tumblr. J Homosex 66(12):1715–1735, 2019 30235077

Charmaraman L, Hodes R, Richer AM: Young sexual minority adolescent experi-ences of self-expression and isolation on social media: cross-sectional survey study. JMIR Ment Health 8(9):e26207, 2021 34524107

Charmaraman L, Hernandez JM, Hodes R: Marginalized and understudied popu-lations using digital media, in Handbook of Adolescent Digital Media Use and Mental Health. Edited by Jacqueline N, Telzer EH, Prinstein MJ. New York, Cam-bridge University Press, 2022, pp 188–213

Christensen MA: "Tindersluts" and "Tinderellas": examining the digital affordances shaping the (hetero)sexual scripts of young womxn on Tinder. Sociological Per-spectives 64(3):432–449, 2021

Cooper RM, Blumenfeld WJ: Responses to cyberbullying: a descriptive analysis of the frequency of and impact on LGBT and allied youth. J LGBT Youth 9(2):153–177, 2012

Cooper K, Quayle E, Jonsson L, et al: Adolescents and self-taken sexual images: a review of the literature. Comput Human Behav 55:706–716, 2016

Donevan M, Mattebo M: The relationship between frequent pornography con-sumption, behaviours, and sexual preoccupancy among male adolescents in Sweden. Sex Reprod Healthc 12:82–87, 2017 28477937

Duguay S: Dressing up Tinderella: interrogating authenticity claims on the mobile dating app Tinder. Inf Commun Soc 20(3):351–367, 2017

Ellyson AM, Adhia A, Lyons VH, et al: Prevalence, age of initiation, and patterns of co-occurrence of digital dating abuse behaviors nationwide. Child Youth Serv Rev 122:105921, 2021 33776176

Englander E: Low Risk Associated With Most Teenage Sexting: A Study of 617 18-Year-Olds. Bridgewater, MA, MARC Research Reports, 2012. Available at: https://vc.bridgew.edu/marc_reports/6. Accessed November 20, 2023.

Erevik EK, Kristensen JH, Torsheim T, et al: Tinder use and romantic relationship formations: a large-scale longitudinal study. Front Psychol 11:1757, 2020 32922327

Finkelhor D, Turner H, Colburn D: Prevalence of online sexual offenses against chil-dren in the US. JAMA Netw Open 5(10):e2234471–e2234471, 2022 36239942

Fritz N, Paul B: From orgasms to spanking: a content analysis of the agentic and ob-jectifying sexual scripts in feminist, for women, and mainstream pornography. Sex Roles 77(9–10):639–652, 2017

Galovan AM, Drouin M, McDaniel BT: Sexting profiles in the United States and Canada: implications for individual and relationship well-being. Comput Human Behav 79:19–29, 2018

Garcia JR, Gesselman AN, Siliman SA, et al: Sexting among singles in the USA: prevalence of sending, receiving, and sharing sexual messages and images. Sex Health 13:428–435, 2016 27470210

Hardy SA, Hurst JL, Price J, et al: The socialization of attitudes about sex and their role in adolescent pornography use. J Adolesc 72:70–82, 2019 30856421

Herbenick D, Fu T-C, Wright P, et al: Diverse sexual behaviors and pornography use: findings from a nationally representative probability survey of Americans aged 18 to 60 years. J Sex Med 17(4):623–633, 2020 32081698

Howard DE, Debnam KJ, Strausser A: "I'm a stalker and proud of it": adolescent girls' perceptions of the mixed utilities associated with internet and social networking use in their dating relationships. Youth Soc 51(6):773–792, 2019

Keles B, McCrae N, Grealish A: A systematic review: the influence of social media on depression, anxiety and psychological distress in adolescents. Int J Adolesc Youth 25(1):79–93, 2020

Klein V, Šević S, Kohut T, et al: Longitudinal assessment of the association between the use of sexually explicit material, hyperfemininity, and sexual agency in adolescent women. Psychol Sex 13(2):213–227, 2020

Lippman JR, Campbell SW: Damned if you do, damned if you don't…if you're a girl: relational and normative contexts of adolescent sexting in the United States. J Child Media 8(4):371–386, 2014

Lofgren-Mårtenson L, Månsson S-A: Lust, love, and life: a qualitative study of Swedish adolescents' perceptions and experiences with pornography. J Sex Res 47(6):568–579, 2010 19731132

Ma J, Korpak AK, Choukas-Bradley S, et al: Patterns of online relationship seeking among transgender and gender diverse adolescents: advice for others and common inquiries. Psychol Sex Orientat Gend Divers 9(3):287–299, 2022

MacDonald K, Imburgia TM, Auerswald C, et al: Sexting among adolescent urban males. J Adolesc Health 62(2):S126, 2018

Madigan S, Ly A, Rash CL, et al: Prevalence of multiple forms of sexting behavior among youth: a systematic review and meta-analysis. JAMA Pediatr 172(4):327–335, 2018 29482215

Maes C, Vandenbosch L: Adolescents' use of sexually explicit internet material over the course of 2019–2020 in the context of the COVID-19 pandemic: a three-wave panel study. Arch Sex Behav 51(1):105–121, 2022a 35001225

Maes C, Vandenbosch L: Physically distant, virtually close: adolescents' sexting behaviors during a strict lockdown period of the COVID-19 pandemic. Comput Human Behav 126:107033, 2022b 34608353

Maes C, Schreurs L, van Oosten JMF, et al: #(Me)too much? The role of sexualizing online media in adolescents' resistance towards the MeToo movement and acceptance of rape myths. J Adolesc 77:59–69, 2019 31654849

Maes C, Van Ouytsel J, Vandenbosch L: Victim blaming and non-consensual forwarding of sexts among late adolescents and young adults. Arch Sex Behav 52(4):1767–1783, 2023a 36745284

Maes C, Wright PJ, Vandenbosch L: Adolescents' preference for mainstream and paraphilic pornography and sexual health components: attention to within- and between-person dynamics over time. Health Comm 27:1–13, 2023b 38534989

Marengo D, Settanni M, Longobardi C: The associations between sex drive, sexual self-concept, sexual orientation, and exposure to online victimization in Italian adolescents: investigating the mediating role of verbal and visual sexting behaviors. Child Youth Serv Rev 102:18–26, 2019

Morelli M, Bianchi D, Baiocco R, et al: Sexting, psychological distress and dating violence among adolescents and young adults. Psicothema 28(2):137–142, 2016 27112809

Mori C, Cooke JE, Temple JR, et al: The prevalence of sexting behaviors among emerging adults: a meta-analysis. Arch Sex Behav 49(4):1103–1119, 2020 32072397

Mosley MA, Lancaster M: Affection and abuse: technology use in adolescent romantic relationships. Am J Fam Ther 47(1):52–66, 2019

Palmer NA, Kosciw JG, Greytak EA, et al: Out Online: The Experiences of Lesbian, Gay, Bisexual, and Transgender Youth on the Internet. New York, GLSEN and Center for Innovative Public Health Research, 2013. Available at: https://www.glsen.org/sites/default/files/2020-01/Out_Online_Full_Report_2013.pdf. Accessed November 20, 2023.

Pampati S, Lowry R, Moreno MA, et al: Having a sexual photo shared without permission and associated health risks: a snapshot of nonconsensual sexting. JAMA Pediatr 174(6):618–619, 2020 32202601

Peter J, Valkenburg PM: Adolescents' use of sexually explicit internet material and sexual uncertainty: the role of involvement and gender. Commun Monogr 77(3):357–375, 2010

Peter J, Valkenburg PM: The use of sexually explicit internet material and its antecedents: a longitudinal comparison of adolescents and adults. Arch Sex Behav 40(5):1015–1025, 2011 20623250

Peter J, Valkenburg PM: Adolescents and pornography: a review of 20 years of research. J Sex Res 53(4–5):509–531, 2016 27105446

Reed L, Conn C, Wachter K: Name-calling, jealousy, and break-ups: teen girls' and boys' worst experiences of digital dating. Child Youth Serv Rev 108:104607, 2020

Rice E, Craddock J, Hemler M, et al: Associations between sexting behaviors and sexual behaviors among mobile phone-owning teens in Los Angeles. Child Dev 89(1):110–117, 2018 28556896

Ringrose J, Harvey L, Gill R, et al: Teen girls, sexual double standards and "sexting": gendered value in digital image exchange. Fem Theory 14(3):305–323, 2013

Robb MB, Mann S: 2022: Teens and Pornography. San Francisco, CA, Common Sense Media, 2023

Romo DL, Garnett C, Younger AP, et al: Social media use and its association with sexual risk and parental monitoring among a primarily Hispanic adolescent population. J Pediatr Adolesc Gynecol 30(4):466–473, 2017 28216129

Sánchez-Jiménez V, Pérez MO, Fernández NM, et al: Cyberdating abuse and sexting in adolescence, in Online Peer Engagement in Adolescence: Positive and Negative Aspects of Online Social Interaction. Edited by Van Zalk N, Monks CP. New York, Routledge/Taylor & Francis Group, 2020, pp 103–121

Thompson L: "I can be your Tinder nightmare": harassment and misogyny in the online sexual marketplace. Fem Psychol 28(1):69–89, 2018

Tienda M, Goldberg RE, Westreich JR: Adolescents' partner search in the digital age: correlates and characteristics of relationships initiated online. J Youth Adolesc 51(3):393–408, 2022 35066707

van Oosten JM: Sexually explicit internet material and adolescents' sexual uncertainty: the role of disposition-content congruency. Arch Sex Behav 45(4):1011–1022, 2016 26373650

Van Ouytsel J, Walrave M, Ponnet K: Sexting within adolescents' romantic relationships: how is it related to perceptions of love and verbal conflict? Comput Human Behav 97:216–221, 2019

Van Ouytsel J, Walrave M, De Marez L, et al: A first investigation into gender minority adolescents' sexting experiences. J Adolesc 84:213–218, 2020 33007516

Wachs S, Wright MF, Gámez-Guadix M, et al: How are consensual, non-consensual, and pressured sexting linked to depression and self-harm? The moderating effects of demographic variables. Int J Environ Res Public Health 18(5):2597, 2021 33807667

Walker K, Sleath E: A systematic review of the current knowledge regarding revenge pornography and non-consensual sharing of sexually explicit media. Aggress Violent Behav 36:9–24, 2017

Weinstein E, James C: Behind Their Screens: What Teens Are Facing (and Adults Are Missing). Cambridge, MA, MIT Press, 2022

Wolak J, Finkelhor D, Walsh W, et al: Sextortion of minors: characteristics and dynamics. J Adolesc Health 62(1):72–79, 2018 29055647

Wright PJ: Pornography and the sexual socialization of children: current knowledge and a theoretical future. J Child Media 8(3):305–312, 2014

Wright PJ, Tokunaga RS, Kraus A, et al: Pornography consumption and satisfaction: a meta-analysis. Hum Commun Res 43(3):315–343, 2017

Wright PJ, Paul B, Herbenick D: Pornography, impersonal sex, and sexual aggression: a test of the confluence model in a national probability sample of men in the U.S. Aggress Behav 47(5):593–602, 2021 34076267

3

Dignity, Diversity, and the Challenges of Bullying and Hateful Speech

Susan M. Swearer, Ph.D., L.P.
Catherine M. Carney, M.A.
Jared S. Noetzel, M.A.
Amanda R. Barrett, B.S.

Bullying is a ubiquitous problem across the globe that impacts people of all ages and nationalities (National Academies of Sciences, Engineering, and Medicine 2016). More than four decades of research has studied the causes, correlates, and consequences of involvement in bullying, and yet, although we understand the complexities underlying this intractable behavior, solving the problem of bullying remains a challenge (Swearer and Hymel 2015). In this chapter, we explore bullying and hateful speech from the perspectives of dignity and diversity. Embracing diversity is vital for a healthy society; however, most societies struggle with discrimination, bullying, and hateful speech online as well as offline. The need to balance the value of freedom of speech with dignity for all persons is the nexus between bullying and prosocial behavior. We assert that respecting the dignity of all persons and treating everyone with kindness are key for mitigating bullying. Throughout this chapter we also highlight youth voices; the deidentified quotes are from youth participants in an individualized cognitive-behavioral intervention for bullying involvement called the Target Bullying Intervention Program (T-BIP; Swearer et al. 2014).

Defining Bullying

Bullying is a complex behavior that occurs both in person and online and is embedded within broader social and cultural contexts. The most widely accepted definition was developed by Olweus (1993) and later adopted by the Centers for Disease Control and Prevention (CDC; Gladden et al. 2014) and describes *bullying* as unwanted harmful behavior characterized by intentionality, repetition or the likelihood of repetition, and an imbalance of power between the perpetrator and victim. Bullying may involve direct (i.e., face-to-face interactions) or indirect behaviors, which can be further classified as physical, verbal, relational, or electronic bullying. Youth can be involved in this dynamic by bullying others, being bullied, observing bullying, or some combination of these roles. Participation in bullying occurs along a continuum in which youth may play multiple roles that change across time and settings (Espelage and Swearer 2003).

Social Ecology of Bullying Involvement

Youth interact across a number of contexts throughout their development. Bronfenbrenner's (1977) social ecological theory posits that development and behaviors are shaped and influenced by the interactions between an individual and the systems that impact their life, ranging from proximal influences (e.g., peers, family, school) to more distal influences and broader systems (e.g., neighborhood, culture, social norms). To understand bullying, we must first understand the developmental contexts that facilitate and attenuate these behaviors and their effects (Swearer and Hymel 2015). Two significant contexts impacting young people and their interactions include the school setting and online platforms such as social media.

Schools, as the place where youth spend most of their day, are important settings for bullying behaviors. Bullying occurs in multiple areas both inside and outside of school, ranging from the school building (e.g., classroom, lunchroom, bathroom) to the wider school grounds (e.g., playground or school bus). It is most likely to occur in physical spaces where there is less adult supervision, such as hallways and playgrounds (Smokowski and Kopasz 2005). Furthermore, it is more likely to occur and to be socially reinforced in schools where aggression is prevalent and normative (Jackson et al. 2015; Sentse et al. 2015). *Cyberbullying*, or bullying on online platforms, is a rising concern for school personnel given the increase in available technology and increased access to social media platforms among school-age youth (Kowalski et al. 2019; Selkie et al. 2016).

The online environment extends and reinforces offline relationships and social processes because significant overlap exists between interactions in school contexts and those on social media (Boyd 2014). Social media can be used for positive behaviors, such as community building, activism, sharing narratives, socializing, or self-expression (Boyd 2014). However, its accessibility, publicity, and potential for anonymity also make it a prime context in which harmful behaviors can be fostered and promoted. Unlike in-person bullying, cyberbullying does not cease when the school day ends and may persist indefinitely until the perpetrator decides to stop (Estévez et al. 2020). The audience for cyberbullying may also be larger, with the possibility for permanency, availability of multiple settings (i.e., bullying across different platforms, such as TikTok, Instagram, gaming platforms), and wide distribution through sharing. Moreover, social media interactions can be asynchronous, which may increase the likelihood of experiencing ruminative thoughts because individuals can review the post repeatedly over time (Hamilton et al. 2021).

> Kaleah, an eighth grade student, said that she was bullied in seventh grade through texting and saw others being bullied online by having "mean things" written about them. She shared that being bullied made her feel sick and sad. When talking about cyberbullying and social media, Kaleah stated, "you have all the time in the world to do the bullying and talk about others."

Prevalence of Bullying Involvement Across Development

Bullying occurs at all ages, but the consensus is that bullying behaviors peak during middle school and then decrease with age (Nansel et al. 2001; Pellegrini and Bartini 2000). This period is a critical time in adolescence during which youth may be exploring their identities and navigating new social roles and groups (Pellegrini and Long 2002). Bullying involvement also varies by type, with studies demonstrating that physical bullying is more common during elementary school but declines into adolescence (Wang et al. 2012; Zych et al. 2020). Conversely, indirect patterns of aggression (i.e., social and relational bullying) increase during adolescence (Smith and Gross 2008). Together, these findings demonstrate that bullying is common across all ages but is most prevalent during early adolescence, when social groups are renegotiated and changes in the school environment may lead to a reestablishment of social roles within the peer group.

Sam, an eighth grade student, told us that he was bullied when he started middle school. He said, "most of the sixth graders got bullied because we were at the bottom of the food chain. But now that I'm in eighth grade, I bully the sixth graders. It's just what we do at my school."

In addition to age, sex and gender[1] also influence the form and extent of bullying behaviors. Overall, males are more likely to be involved in bullying, both as perpetrators and victims, compared with females (Carbone-Lopez et al. 2010; Nansel et al. 2001; Pellegrini and Long 2002). A meta-analysis of cyberbullying research found that sex differences persisted in cyberbullying involvement, with males more likely to be perpetrators of cyberbullying (Sun et al. 2016). As perpetrators, males are more likely to use direct forms of aggression, whereas females are more likely to engage in indirect bullying (Carbone-Lopez et al. 2010; Farrington and Baldry 2010).

Estimates of prevalence rates have found that approximately one-third of school-age youth report involvement in face-to-face bullying as either a perpetrator or a victim (Modecki et al. 2014; Zych et al. 2015). Among U.S. adolescents ages 12–18 years, approximately one in five (20.2%) reported being bullied (National Center for Education Statistics 2019). Estimations of bullying perpetration range from 5% to 13% among youth (Hymel and Swearer 2015), while estimates for involvement in both roles (i.e., as a bully and as a victim) range from 2% to 11.5% (Dulmus et al. 2006; Yang and Salmivalli 2013). Studies examining the prevalence of cyberbullying indicate that approximately one in four students will experience it as a victim (Li 2006; Wright et al. 2009), with estimates ranging from 6% to 30% (Kowalski et al. 2014; Patchin and Hinduja 2012). Approximately one in six students has participated in cyberbullying behaviors (Li 2006; Wright et al. 2009).

The prevalence of traditional bullying and that of cyberbullying cannot be examined in isolation, however, because offline and online behaviors overlap in most youth's lives. Youth who are bullied at school are more likely to be bullied online, and those bullied online are more likely to bully others at school (Kowalski et al. 2014; Lazuras et al. 2017; Myers et al. 2017; Waasdorp and Bradshaw 2015), which shows how contexts that normalize aggression can increase bullying behaviors. In a meta-analysis synthesizing findings from 80 studies, traditional bullying and cyberbullying were found

---

[1] Within the referenced literature, there is significant variation on the operationalization of sex and/or gender (e.g., some studies referring to a binary conceptualization of gender [boy/girl] and some using *gender* and *sex* interchangeably); therefore, this chapter refers to this construct unidimensionally as "sex and gender."

to be moderately correlated, with higher degrees of association between per-petration than victimization. However, this co-occurrence was particularly robust for both roles when relational bullying was examined specifically (Modecki et al. 2014). It is important to note that these rates of bullying in-volvement are higher for youth who belong to marginalized groups and may be exposed to identity-based bullying, online hate, or hateful speech (Kan-sok-Dusche et al. 2023).

Identity-based bullying, also known as bias-based bullying, involves tar-geting someone on the basis of their identity or group membership. Studies have shown that youth from cultural, ethnic, or sexual minority groups are at increased risk for cybervictimization (Espinoza and Wright 2018). For example, LGBTQ+ youth are more likely to be victimized than their straight, cisgender peers (Clark et al. 2014; National Academy of Medicine 2011). Racial and ethnic minority youth, as well as immigrant youth, also experi-ence more identity-based bullying, and this is exacerbated by their minori-tized status (Durkin et al. 2012). Other identity factors, such as disability status, have also been associated with increased risk for bullying victimiza-tion when compared with nondisabled peers (Bear et al. 2015).

There is limited literature on the experiences and impacts of cyberbul-lying across people with intersecting identities (e.g., a White, able-bodied gay male or a Black, disabled, straight, gender-nonconforming person). One study found sex differences in reported cyberbullying victimization among White youth, with females reporting higher victimization; however, this dif-ference was not found among the non-White sample (Stoll and Block 2015, cited in Espinoza and Wright 2018). A study by Angoff and Barnhart (2021) demonstrated that, overall, sexual and/or gender minority (SGM) youth were more likely to be victims of both in-person and online bullying, with bisexual youth having higher cyberbullying victimization rates compared with other sexual minority youth. This study also revealed that racially mi-noritized youth experienced lower rates of bullying; however, this effect was only found among heterosexual youth. These findings show that generaliza-tions about prevalence rates across demographic groups may fail to consider nuances of intersectionality and the broader social norms related to youth identity, underscoring the need for targeted interventions that address in-tersectionality (Angoff and Barnhart 2021).

Understanding Social Media and Bullying

Given the high degree of overlap and continuity between in-person and on-line bullying behaviors, much of the research on cyberbullying stems from what we know about traditional bullying. However, cyberbullying has also been conceptualized and treated as an online safety issue, with attempts to address safety concerns via social media policies (Milosevic 2018). More recent approaches have begun to emphasize the societal values, social norms, and group processes that encourage and maintain aggressive behaviors, such as hateful speech and cyberbullying. Critical to this conceptualization is understanding 1) how youth view themselves in relation to others and 2) how these processes are shaped by societal pressures and messages about how to attain status and worth.

The Power of Anonymity

In examining risk factors unique to cyberbullying, some researchers have postulated that anonymity may play a role in the initiation and maintenance of online bullying behaviors (Barlett 2015a). Social media platforms allow users to experiment with different identities, often under the guise of an anonymous username. This anonymity protects the user from negative evaluations or social repercussions (Barlett 2015a; Barlett and Gentile 2012), leading to greater disinhibition of behavior. As a result, youth may be more likely to say or do things that they would not otherwise say or do in person. Researchers have suggested that this anonymity, or the perception thereof, is a prominent characteristic that helps distinguish cyberbullying from traditional bullying (Li 2007; Smith et al. 2008) and may help explain why cybervictimization is likely to be perceived as more severe than traditional bullying victimization by youth who have been bullied online (Slonje et al. 2013; Sticca and Perren 2013).

Research has found that 29% of adolescents who have experienced cyberbullying did not know the identity of their aggressor (Patchin and Hinduja 2006). Other studies found higher rates in which most of the victimized youth did not know who bullied them (Kowalski and Limber 2007; Li 2007). Perceived anonymity has been found to predict both greater frequency of cyberbullying behaviors and positive attitudes toward cyberbullying (Barlett 2015a, 2015b; Barlett and Gentile 2012). Central to this relationship is the ability to harm others while avoiding real-world consequences (Mishna et al. 2009).

> Omar, a fourth grade student, has been bullied since kindergarten and eventually began bullying to defend himself from other students. He described a situation on the online video game platform Roblox when another player "called me mean names and said he didn't want to keep playing with me." He stated, "I felt sad and confused about who was leaving me out and why."

Influence of Social Norms

Efforts have been made to understand bullying by recognizing and evaluating the broader norms and values that shape social interactions (Hong and Espelage 2012; Maunder and Crafter 2018; Salmivalli 2010; Swearer and Hymel 2015). In line with this social-ecological approach, bullying has been reconceptualized as a violation of human rights, with roots in broader social values that normalize using aggression to obtain status and dignity within the social group (Milosevic et al. 2022; Søndergaard 2012). Indeed, growing evidence indicates that bullying may be a goal-oriented strategy used to obtain social status, power, and popularity (Faris and Felmlee 2014; Salmivalli 2010; Samson et al. 2022; Volk et al. 2014).

Dignity should be understood as innate to all people and, unlike respect, should not have to be earned; however, societal norms perpetuate the belief that worth and social status are gained from external sources, namely others' approval (Milosevic et al. 2022; Søndergaard 2012). Adolescents are likely to believe that their worth derives from their ability to establish acceptance within a social group and depends on others' evaluations and validation (Skymba et al. 2022; Xu et al. 2022). Thus, dignity theory is an important heuristic for understanding and mitigating bullying behavior.

Motivated by the need to belong, fear of exclusion, and desire for social status, bullying and cyberbullying can be understood as social processes that result from feelings of social insecurity (Søndergaard 2012). Consistent with this perspective, relationships between bullying behaviors and social status (i.e., popularity) have been well established in the literature. Bullying has been found to be motivated by attempts to earn social approval and gain status or membership within a group (Salmivalli 2010; Witvliet et al. 2010) and is more likely to occur when aggression is normalized by the group (Salmivalli and Voeten 2004). Furthermore, popularity has been found to be positively associated with bullying involvement (de Bruyn et al. 2010; Witvliet et al. 2010), and this relationship is particularly salient for adolescents, who are more likely to use bullying as a tool to obtain popularity and social status among their peers (Duffy et al. 2017; Juvonen and Galván 2008; Ojanen and Findley-Van Nostrand 2014; Thornberg 2015).

When applied to the online context, messages of worth that are based on external attributes are common. Adolescents may seek social validation via the number of likes, shares, comments, views, or followers/friends that they receive, which has important implications for self-esteem and self-worth (Meeus et al. 2019). In line with these notions, studies have found that adolescents are more likely to present idealized versions of themselves online in an attempt to obtain peer validation (Throuvala et al. 2019; Yau and Reich 2019). Similarly, a positive association between engagement in cyberbullying behaviors, popularity (Wegge et al. 2016; Wright et al. 2022), and group affiliation (Solomontos-Kountouri and Strohmeier 2021) has been found among adolescents.

> Francesca, a sixth grader, said that she has been bullied by her friends and has seen others being bullied online or via texting. When discussing cyberbullying and bullying via social media, she shared, "followers give people power on social media."

At a group level, bullying may be used to reinforce or maintain group status and membership at the expense of members of other groups (i.e., "in-group" vs. "out-group" interactions) (Jones et al. 2009; Ojala and Nesdale 2004). Such group-level processes may underlie identity-based bullying behaviors and hateful speech, whereby membership in one group is framed as holding more social power and status, while the welfare and dignity of members of the other group are targeted based on their identity or group membership. Together, research suggests, aggressive behaviors are often used as a tool to obtain social status and affiliation, both in person and online. Dignity theory suggests that aggressive behaviors are reinforced through the attainment of social status or attention due to the belief that worth must be obtained through external validation, often in the form of likes, shares, follows, or comments on social media platforms.

> Camryn, a seventh grader, was involved in the bullying dynamic by being bullied, bullying others, and witnessing bullying. She described that she bullied others because that's "what my friends did" and that bullying was a way for her to gain "power through popularity." Camryn shared that popular kids at her school bully others or "go along with it because that's what others are doing."

Minority Stress Theory and Cyberbullying

Minority stress theory posits that individuals from marginalized groups experience unique and chronic stressors based on their identity, such as bullying, harassment, and discrimination (Meyer 2003). This theory has been used to understand disparities in mental and physical health, as well as academic and social outcomes, for SGM individuals (Meyer 2003); however, it has been applied to other identities in recent years, including race, disability status, and their intersections (Cyrus 2017; Hayes et al. 2011; Lund 2021). Cyberbullying experiences differ across race, sex/gender, LGBTQ+ identity, disability status, and the presence of multiple intersecting identities. According to minority stress theory, bullying and cyberbullying constitute external stressors that increase the risk for negative psychosocial outcomes.

Weinstein et al. (2021) focused on racially targeted discrimination and cyberbullying and found a co-occurrence over time of the amount of time spent online and the experience of racial discrimination, both on- and offline. Specifically, earlier experiences of bullying victimization were predictive of victimization online and racially targeted discrimination offline. Similarly, Thomas et al. (2022) investigated the influence of online racial discrimination in a sample of Black and Hispanic youth and found that social media use alone was not related to depressive and anxious symptoms; however, their relationship was mediated by both individual and "vicarious [indirect]" racial discrimination.

SGM youth also face unique stressors related to cyberbullying. Generally, research supports that SGM youth are significantly more likely to be victims of bullying, cyberbullying, and co-occurring (in-person and online) bullying (Ash-Houchen and Lo 2018; Myers et al. 2017). In accordance with minority stress theory, research has demonstrated more severe impacts of cyberbullying for SGM youth. For example, one study found that suicidal ideation was highest for sexual minority youth who were victims of bullying, with no effects found for ethnicity or gender (Mueller et al. 2015). Often, this bullying is based on the perception of the victim being an SGM, especially in cases of cyberbullying. One student reported that "someone in my old school...acted stereotypically gay, but no one ever knew if he really was, but all the guys would make fun of him and say he was gay...on Facebook using words like 'fag' and stuff" (Mishna et al. 2020).

Like SGM youth, youth with disabilities reported higher cyberbullying victimization compared with nondisabled youth (Kowalski and Toth 2017). A systematic review of individuals with autism spectrum disorder experiencing different forms of interpersonal violence, including bullying and cyberbullying, found that although victimization rates were higher for autistic compared with allistic (i.e., not autistic) individuals, victimization rates were even higher for autistic individuals who were also members of other minority groups (Cooke et al. 2022). Kowalski and Toth (2017) found that among participants in the age range their study investigated (16–20 years), disability was not a predictor of significantly worse outcomes from cyberbullying victimization compared with nondisabled peers. However, a similar study among college students found that disabled participants reported significantly worse outcomes from cyberbullying, such as higher depression and lower self-esteem, when compared with nondisabled victims, which suggests that more research should be done to investigate these impacts (Kowalski et al. 2016).

> Mitchell, an eighth grader, said that his peers have called him names, made fun of him, written mean things about him online, and said mean things behind his back. He stated that "other kids think I'm annoying because I have autism." He also shared that he has witnessed his friends being bullied "because they are different and LGBTQ." Mitchell reported, "Victims have a hard time getting the problem to stop. It's a lose-lose situation, because they get called a snitch if they tell a teacher and, if they don't tell, the bullying won't stop."

This idea of youth being "different" is frequently cited as the main reason for both traditional and online bullying. When this occurs on the basis of identity and is normalized by broader group and social norms, youth experience worse outcomes. Critical to mitigating the effects of minority stress on bullying outcomes is the need to address aggression as a tool used by youth for obtaining status and worth and to explicitly address the reasons underlying the function of bullying behavior.

Bullying and Mental Health

Bullying victimization and perpetration have been recognized as important public health concerns (Feder 2007) that contribute to serious and long-lasting psychosocial problems. Studies have consistently documented the relationship between bullying and internalizing and externalizing problems, both as predictors and outcomes of bullying involvement (Gladden et al. 2014; Moore et al. 2017). Regardless of their role, youth who are involved in the bullying dynamic are at greater risk for depressive and anxious symptoms and conduct problems (Arslan et al. 2021; Eastman et al. 2018). Moreover, youth who bully others or experience bullying in person are at an increased risk for negative outcomes later in life, including lower academic achievement, poorer health, increased drug use, and greater internalizing symptoms and behavioral problems (Arslan et al. 2021; Copeland et al. 2013; Sigurdson et al. 2014).

Studies investigating the impact of cyberbullying have found similar adverse outcomes for involved youth; however, some research suggests that cyberbullying may predict unique or exacerbated negative outcomes beyond those of traditional bullying (Giumetti and Kowalski 2016). Cybervictimization is associated with increased odds of externalizing and internalizing symptoms (Waasdorp and Bradshaw 2015), including increased risk for self-harm and suicide attempts, when compared with other forms of traditional bullying (Yang et al. 2021). However, given the high degree of co-occurrence between traditional and cyberbullying, outcomes are likely to represent an additive effect (Landstedt and Persson 2014). Indeed, Jones et al. (2023) recently found that youth who had experienced identity-based bullying exclusively online had fewer negative outcomes than those who experienced identity-based bullying in person; however, when bullying was persistent across online and in-person settings, it was associated with the greatest degree of distress for youth. These findings point to the importance of assessing for and addressing bullying experiences that occur across settings and emphasize the need for intervention with youth who experience victimization both in person and online.

> Drew, a sixth grader who was referred to the T-BIP intervention for physical and verbal bullying behaviors, endorsed clinically significant levels of depressive symptoms. He shared that he has had thoughts about "what the world would be like without me" for multiple years, and these feelings worsened when he was bullied.

Mitigating Bullying Behavior Through Mental Wellness

To mitigate bullying behaviors, students must be taught and modeled social-emotional skills and how to treat others with dignity and respect. Examples in this chapter from the T-BIP illustrate how an individualized cognitive-behavioral intervention can help uncover the function of the behavior and mitigate bullying behaviors. Another concrete mitigation strategy is teaching kindness. Lady Gaga's Born This Way Foundation recently launched a new program, #BeKind365, which is a social media tool designed to promote kindness. The Born This Way Foundation offers a free website, Be Kind 365 (https://bekind365.world), centered around promoting kindness. After creating an account, students can interact with the site in various ways to receive a "building block" that counts toward their progress in the Kind Connector, a virtual showcase of kind acts occurring around the globe. Like teaching kindness, teaching and modeling prosocial behaviors is critical for mitigating bullying.

> Mark, a ninth grader, was referred to T-BIP for targeting a peer online. He demonstrated difficulty identifying how his behaviors affected his peers, stating that he believed that "growing up without the bullying will make you egotistical." On the assessments, Mark endorsed that it was difficult for him to see things from another person's point of view and that he is not usually bothered by other people's problems. During the T-BIP, he practiced cogni-

tive challenging and perspective-taking skills. At the end of the intervention session, Mark said that he "learned about the opposite view" of bullying and that it was helpful.

A middle school counselor referred two students to the T-BIP and shared, "We have had a few other sixth graders recently use T-BIP, and to say that it's life-changing is an understatement. The assessment is extensive (4 hours), but each student I've had says it flies by and is extremely helpful…. Now that I've had a few students go through it, I can speak more to what it is and how much it can help a student."

A healthy community is created by the people in that community, and it is everyone's responsibility to model healthy behavior and to set clear expectations that everyone deserves to be treated with dignity and respect. When this happens, bullying and cyberbullying will not be normative behaviors. However, given the decades of research on these behaviors and the intractable nature of bullying, we know there is much work to be done.

References

Angoff HD, Barnhart WR: Bullying and cyberbullying among LGBQ and heterosexual youth from an intersectional perspective: findings from the 2017 National Youth Risk Behavior Survey. J Sch Violence 20(3):274–286, 2021

Arslan G, Allen K-A, Tanhan A: School bullying, mental health, and wellbeing in adolescents: mediating impact of positive psychological orientations. Child Indic Res 14(3):1007–1026, 2021

Ash-Houchen W, Lo CC: Intersections of gender and sexual minority status: co-occurring bullying victimization among adolescents. Comput Human Behav 80:262–270, 2018

Barlett CP: Anonymously hurting others online: the effect of anonymity on cyberbullying frequency. Psychol Pop Media Cult 4(2):70–79, 2015a

Barlett CP: Predicting adolescent's cyberbullying behavior: a longitudinal risk analysis. J Adolesc 41:86–95, 2015b 25828551

Barlett CP, Gentile DA: Attacking others online: the formation of cyberbullying in late adolescence. Psychol Pop Media Cult 1(2):123–135, 2012

Bear GG, Mantz LS, Glutting JJ, et al: Differences in bullying victimization between students with and without disabilities. School Psych Rev 44(1):98–116, 2015

Boyd D: It's Complicated: The Social Lives of Networked Teens. New Haven, CT, Yale University Press, 2014

Bronfenbrenner U: Toward an experimental ecology of human development. Am Psychol 32(7):513–531, 1977

Carbone-Lopez K, Esbensen F-A, Brick BT: Correlates and consequences of peer victimization: gender differences in direct and indirect forms of bullying. Youth Violence Juv Justice 8(4):332–350, 2010

Clark TC, Lucassen MFG, Bullen P, et al: The health and well-being of transgender high school students: results from the New Zealand adolescent health survey (Youth '12). J Adolesc Health 55(1):93–99, 2014 24438852

Cooke K, Ridgway K, Westrupp E, et al: The Prevalence and Risk Factors of Autistic Experiences of Interpersonal Violence: A Systematic Review and Meta-Analysis. Durham, NC, Research Square, November 23, 2022. Available at: https://www.researchsquare.com/article/rs-2286120/v1. Accessed November 20, 2023.

Copeland WE, Wolke D, Angold A, et al: Adult psychiatric outcomes of bullying and being bullied by peers in childhood and adolescence. JAMA Psychiatry 70(4):419–426, 2013 23426798

Cyrus K: Multiple minorities as multiply marginalized: applying the minority stress theory to LGBTQ people of color. J Gay Lesbian Ment Health 21(3):194–202, 2017

de Bruyn EH, Cillessen AHN, Wissink IB: Associations of peer acceptance and perceived popularity with bullying and victimization in early adolescence. J Early Adolesc 30(4):543–566, 2010

Duffy AL, Penn S, Nesdale D, et al: Popularity: does it magnify associations between popularity prioritization and the bullying and defending behavior of early adolescent boys and girls? Soc Dev 26(2):263–277, 2017

Dulmus C, Sowers K, Theriot M: Prevalence and bullying experiences of victims and victims who become bullies (bully victims) at rural schools. Vict Offenders 1:15–31, 2006

Durkin K, Hunter S, Levin KA, et al: Discriminatory peer aggression among children as a function of minority status and group proportion in school context. Eur J Soc Psychol 42(2):243–251, 2012

Eastman M, Foshee V, Ennett S, et al: Profiles of internalizing and externalizing symptoms associated with bullying victimization. J Adolesc 65:101–110, 2018 29573643

Espelage D, Swearer S: Research on school bullying and victimization: what have we learned and where do we go from here? School Psych Rev 32:365–383, 2003

Espinoza G, Wright M: Cyberbullying experiences among marginalized youth: what do we know and where do we go next? J Child Adolesc Trauma 11(1):1–5, 2018 32318132

Estévez E, Cañas E, Estévez JF, et al: Continuity and overlap of roles in victims and aggressors of bullying and cyberbullying in adolescence: a systematic review. Int J Environ Res Public Health 17(20):20, 2020 33066202

Faris R, Felmlee D: Casualties of social combat: school networks of peer victimization and their consequences. Am Sociol Rev 79:228–257, 2014

Farrington DP, Baldry AC: Individual risk factors for school bullying. J Aggress Conflict Peace Res 2:4–16, 2010

Feder L: Bullying as a public health issue. Int J Offender Ther Comp Criminol 51(5):491–494, 2007 17848710

Giumetti GW, Kowalski RM: Cyberbullying matters: examining the incremental impact of cyberbullying on outcomes over and above traditional bullying in North America, in Cyberbullying Across the Globe. Edited by Navarro R, Yubero S, Larrañaga E. Cham, Switzerland, Springer, 2016, pp 117–130

Gladden RM, Vivolo-Kantor AM, Hamburger ME, et al: Bullying Surveillance Among Youths: Uniform Definitions for Public Health and Recommended Data Elements, Version 1.0. Atlanta, GA, National Center for Injury Prevention and Control, Centers for Disease Control and Prevention, U.S. Department of Education, 2014. Available at: https://www.cdc.gov/violenceprevention/pdf/bullying-definitions-final-a.pdf. Accessed November 20, 2023.

Hamilton JL, Do QB, Choukas-Bradley S, et al: Where it hurts the most: peer interactions on social media and in person are differentially associated with emotional reactivity and sustained affect among adolescent girls. Res Child Adolesc Psychopathol 49(2):155–167, 2021

Hayes JA, Chun-Kennedy C, Edens A, et al: Do double minority students face double jeopardy? Testing minority stress theory. J Coll Couns 14(2):117–126, 2011

Hong JS, Espelage DL: A review of research on bullying and peer victimization in school: an ecological system analysis. Aggress Violent Behav 17(4):311–322, 2012

Hymel S, Swearer SM: Four decades of research on school bullying: an introduction. Am Psychol 70(4):293–299, 2015 25961310

Jackson DR, Cappella E, Neal JW: Aggression norms in the classroom social network: contexts of aggressive behavior and social preference in middle childhood. Am J Community Psychol 56(3–4):293–306, 2015 26415598

Jones SE, Manstead ASR, Livingstone A: Birds of a feather bully together: group processes and children's responses to bullying. Br J Dev Psychol 27(Pt 4):853–873, 2009 19994483

Jones LM, Montagut AS, Mitchell KJ, et al: Youth bias-based victimization: comparing online only, in-person only, and mixed online/in-person incidents. Int J Bullying Prev 38(19–20), 2023

Juvonen J, Galván A: Peer influence in involuntary social groups: lessons from research on bullying, in Understanding Peer Influence in Children and Adolescents. Edited by Prinstein MJ, Dodge KA. New York, Guilford, 2008, pp 225–244

Kansok-Dusche J, Ballaschk C, Krause N, et al: A systematic review on hate speech among children and adolescents: definitions, prevalence, and overlap with related phenomena. Trauma Violence Abuse 24(4):2598–2615, 2023 35731198

Kowalski RM, Limber SP: Electronic bullying among middle school students. J Adolesc Health 41(6)(Suppl 1):S22–S30, 2007 18047942

Kowalski RM, Toth A: Cyberbullying among youth with and without disabilities. J Child Adolesc Trauma 11(1):7–15, 2017 32318133

Kowalski RM, Giumetti GW, Schroeder AN, et al: Bullying in the digital age: a critical review and meta-analysis of cyberbullying research among youth. Psychol Bull 140(4):1073–1137, 2014 24512111

Kowalski RM, Morgan CA, Drake-Lavelle K, et al: Cyberbullying among college students with disabilities. Comput Human Behav 57:416–427, 2016

Kowalski RM, Limber SP, McCord A: A developmental approach to cyberbullying: prevalence and protective factors. Aggress Violent Behav 45:20–32, 2019

Landstedt E, Persson S: Bullying, cyberbullying, and mental health in young people. Scand J Public Health 42(4):393–399, 2014 24608094

Lazuras L, Barkoukis V, Tsorbatzoudis H: Face-to-face bullying and cyberbullying in adolescents: trans-contextual effects and role overlap. Technol Soc 48:97–101, 2017

Li Q: Cyberbullying in schools: a research of gender differences. Sch Psychol Int 27:157–170, 2006

Li Q: New bottle but old wine: a research of cyberbullying in schools. Comput Human Behav 23(4):1777–1791, 2007

Lund EM: Examining the potential applicability of the minority stress model for explaining suicidality in individuals with disabilities. Rehabil Psychol 66(2):183–191, 2021 34014712

Maunder RE, Crafter S: School bullying from a sociocultural perspective. Aggress Violent Behav 38:13–20, 2018

Meeus A, Beullens K, Eggermont S: Like me (please?): connecting online self-presentation to pre- and early adolescents' self-esteem. New Media Soc 21(11–12):2386–2403, 2019

Meyer IH: Prejudice, social stress, and mental health in lesbian, gay, and bisexual populations: conceptual issues and research evidence. Psychol Bull 129(5):674–697, 2003 12956539

Milosevic T: Protecting Children Online? Cyberbullying Policies of Social Media Companies. Cambridge, MA, MIT Press, 2018

Milosevic T, Collier A, O'Higgins Norman J: Leveraging dignity theory to understand bullying, cyberbullying, and children's rights. Int J Bullying Prev 4(1):1–5, 2022 35233506

Mishna F, Saini M, Solomon S: Ongoing and online: children and youth's perceptions of cyber bullying. Child Youth Serv Rev 31(12):1222–1228, 2009

Mishna F, Sanders JE, McNeil S, et al: "If Somebody Is Different": a critical analysis of parent, teacher and student perspectives on bullying and cyberbullying. Child Youth Serv Rev 118:105366, 2020

Modecki KL, Minchin J, Harbaugh AG, et al: Bullying prevalence across contexts: a meta-analysis measuring cyber and traditional bullying. J Adolesc Health 55(5):602–611, 2014 25168105

Moore SE, Norman RE, Suetani S, et al: Consequences of bullying victimization in childhood and adolescence: a systematic review and meta-analysis. World J Psychiatry 7(1):60–76, 2017 28401049

Mueller AS, James W, Abrutyn S, et al: Suicide ideation and bullying among US adolescents: examining the intersections of sexual orientation, gender, and race/ethnicity. Am J Public Health 105(5):980–985, 2015 25790421

Myers ZR, Swearer SM, Martin MJ, et al: Cyberbullying and traditional bullying: the experiences of poly victimization among diverse youth. Int J Technoethics 8(2):42–60, 2017

Nansel TR, Overpeck M, Pilla RS, et al: Bullying behaviors among US youth: prevalence and association with psychosocial adjustment. JAMA 285(16):2094–2100, 2001 11311098

National Academies of Sciences, Engineering, and Medicine: Preventing Bullying Through Science, Policy, and Practice. Washington, DC, National Academies Press, 2016

National Academy of Medicine: The Health of Lesbian, Gay, Bisexual, and Transgender People: Building a Foundation for Better Understanding. Washington, DC, National Academies Press, 2011

National Center for Education Statistics: Bullying at School and Electronic Bullying: Condition of Education. U.S. Department of Education, Institute of Education Sciences, 2019

Ojala K, Nesdale D: Bullying and social identity: the effects of group norms and distinctiveness threat on attitudes towards bullying. Br J Dev Psychol 22(1):19–35, 2004

Ojanen T, Findley-Van Nostrand D: Social goals, aggression, peer preference, and popularity: longitudinal links during middle school. Dev Psychol 50(8):2134–2143, 2014 24911564

Olweus D: Bullying at School: What We Know and What We Can Do. Malden, MA, Blackwell Publishing, 1993

Patchin JW, Hinduja S: Bullies move beyond the schoolyard: a preliminary look at cyberbullying. Youth Violence Juv Justice 4(2):148–169, 2006

Patchin JW, Hinduja S: Cyberbullying: an update and synthesis, in Cyberbullying Prevention and Response. Edited by Patchin JW, Hinduja S. New York, Routledge, 2012, pp 12–35

Pellegrini AD, Bartini M: A longitudinal study of bullying, victimization, and peer affiliation during the transition from primary school to middle school. Am Educ Res J 37(3):699–725, 2000

Pellegrini AD, Long JD: A longitudinal study of bullying, dominance, and victimization during the transition from primary school through secondary school. Br J Dev Psychol 20:259–280, 2002

Salmivalli C: Bullying and the peer group: a review. Aggress Violent Behav 15(2):112–120, 2010

Salmivalli C, Voeten M: Connections between attitudes, group norms, and behaviour in bullying situations. Int J Behav Dev 28(3):246–258, 2004

Samson JE, Delgado MA, Louis DF, et al: Bullying and social goal-setting in youth: a meta-analysis. Soc Dev 31(4):945–961, 2022

Selkie EM, Fales JL, Moreno MA: Cyberbullying prevalence among US middle and high school-aged adolescents: a systematic review and quality assessment. J Adolesc Health 58(2):125–133, 2016 26576821

Sentse M, Veenstra R, Kiuru N, et al: A longitudinal multilevel study of individual characteristics and classroom norms in explaining bullying behaviors. J Abnorm Child Psychol 43(5):943–955, 2015 25370007

Sigurdson JF, Wallander J, Sund AM: Is involvement in school bullying associated with general health and psychosocial adjustment outcomes in adulthood? Child Abuse Negl 38(10):1607–1617, 2014 24972719

Skymba HV, Joyce C, Telzer EH, et al: Peer adversity predicts interpersonal needs in adolescent girls. J Res Adolesc 32(4):1566–1579, 2022 35253314

Slonje R, Smith PK, Frisén A: The nature of cyberbullying, and strategies for prevention. Comput Human Behav 29(1):26–32, 2013

Smith RG, Gross AM: Bullying: prevalence and the effect of age and gender. Child Fam Behav Ther 28(4):13–37, 2008

Smith PK, Mahdavi J, Carvalho M, et al: Cyberbullying: its nature and impact in secondary school pupils. J Child Psychol Psychiatry 49(4):376–385, 2008 18363945

Smokowski PR, Kopasz KH: Bullying in school: an overview of types, effects, family characteristics, and intervention strategies. Child Schools 27(2):101–110, 2005

Solomontos-Kountouri O, Strohmeier D: The need to belong as motive for (cyber)bullying and aggressive behavior among immigrant adolescents in Cyprus. New Dir Child Adolesc Dev 2021(177):159–178, 2021 33899327

Søndergaard DM: Bullying and social exclusion anxiety in schools. Br J Sociol Educ 33(3):355–372, 2012

Sticca F, Perren S: Is cyberbullying worse than traditional bullying? Examining the differential roles of medium, publicity, and anonymity for the perceived severity of bullying. J Youth Adolesc 42(5):739–750, 2013 23184483

Stoll LC, Block R Jr: Intersectionality and cyberbullying: a study of cybervictimization in a Midwestern high school. Comput Human Behav 52:387–397, 2015

Sun S, Fan X, Du J: Cyberbullying perpetration: a meta-analysis of gender differences. Int J Internet Sci 11(1):61–81, 2016

Swearer SM, Hymel S: Understanding the psychology of bullying: moving toward a social-ecological diathesis-stress model. Am Psychol 70(4):344–353, 2015 25961315

Swearer SM, Wang C, Collins A, et al: Bullying: a school mental health perspective, in Handbook of School Mental Health, 2nd Edition. Edited by Weist M, Lever NA, Bradshaw CP, et al. New York, Springer, 2014, pp 341–354

Thomas A, Jing M, Chen HY, et al: Taking the good with the bad? Social media and online racial discrimination influences on psychological and academic functioning in Black and Hispanic youth. J Youth Adolesc 52(2):245–257, 2022 36229754

Thornberg R: Distressed bullies, social positioning, and odd victims: young people's explanations of bullying. Child Soc 29(1):15–25, 2015

Throuvala MA, Griffiths MD, Rennoldson M, et al: Motivational processes and dysfunctional mechanisms of social media use among adolescents: a qualitative focus group study. Comput Human Behav 93:164–175, 2019

Volk AA, Dane AV, Marini ZA: What is bullying? A theoretical redefinition. Dev Rev 34(4):327–343, 2014

Waasdorp TE, Bradshaw CP: The overlap between cyberbullying and traditional bullying. J Adolesc Health 56(5):483–488, 2015 25631040

Wang J, Iannotti RJ, Luk JW: Patterns of adolescent bullying behaviors: physical, verbal, exclusion, rumor, and cyber. J Sch Psychol 50(4):521–534, 2012 22710019

Wegge D, Vandebosch H, Eggermont S, et al: Popularity through online harm: the longitudinal associations between cyberbullying and sociometric status in early adolescence. J Early Adolesc 36(1):86–107, 2016

Weinstein M, Jensen MR, Tynes BM: Victimized in many ways: online and offline bullying/harassment and perceived racial discrimination in diverse racial-ethnic minority adolescents. Cultur Divers Ethnic Minor Psychol 27(3):397–407, 2021 34043397

Witvliet M, Olthof T, Hoeksma JB, et al: Peer group affiliation of children: the role of perceived popularity, likeability, and behavioral similarity in bullying. Soc Dev 19(2):285–303, 2010

Wright VH, Burnham JJ, Christopher TI, et al: Cyberbullying: using virtual scenarios to educate and raise awareness. J Comput Teach Educ 26(1):35–42, 2009

Wright MF, Wachs S, Huang Z, et al: Longitudinal associations among Machiavellianism, popularity goals, and adolescents' cyberbullying involvement: the role of gender. J Genet Psychol 183(5):482–493, 2022 35869659

Xu J, Troop-Gordon W, Rudolph KD: Within-person reciprocal associations between peer victimization and need for approval. Dev Psychol 58(10):1999–2011, 2022 35666926

Yang A, Salmivalli C: Different forms of bullying and victimization: bully victims versus bullies and victims. Eur J Dev Psychol 10(6):723–738, 2013

Yang B, Wang B, Sun N, et al: The consequences of cyberbullying and traditional bullying victimization among adolescents: gender differences in psychological symptoms, self-harm and suicidality. Psychiatry Res 306:114219, 2021 34614443

Yau JC, Reich SM: "It's just a lot of work": adolescents' self-presentation norms and practices on Facebook and Instagram. J Res Adolesc 29(1):196–209, 2019 29430759

Zych I, Ortega-Ruiz R, Del Rey R: Systematic review of theoretical studies on bullying and cyberbullying: facts, knowledge, prevention, and intervention. Aggress Violent Behav 23:1–21, 2015

Zych I, Ttofi MM, Llorent VJ, et al: A longitudinal study on stability and transitions among bullying roles. Child Dev 91(2):527–545, 2020 30566232

4

Misinformation, Disinformation, and Mental Health

Sherry Bell, B.A.
Ellen Middaugh, Ph.D.

In this chapter we explore how misinformation impacts the mental health of youth, an area that has received less study than its effects on their physical health. We also discuss the types of information that youth selectively attend to online and why they are susceptible to misinformation in their online spaces.

An *infodemic* has been defined as a wave of information that is broadly and rapidly disseminated. Brought on by the digital era with its proliferation of communication technologies, a tsunami of information has come to include misinformation and disinformation, exposure to which may have adverse effects on youth and their well-being (Rubinelli et al. 2022).

Misinformation is defined as information that is inaccurate, incomplete, or lacks credible evidence (Ha et al. 2021). When created deliberately to mislead audiences, such information is labeled *disinformation* (Ha et al. 2021). The negative impact of misinformation on public health campaign efforts has resulted in associations with heightened anxiety (Freiling et al. 2023), vaccine hesitation (Geana et al. 2021), mistrust in governments (Jennings et al. 2021), and decreased medication adherence (Teplinsky et al. 2022). Recent reports suggest that most misinformation shared on social media is related to political events or coronavirus disease 2019 (COVID-19) (Vosoughi et al. 2018; World Health Organization 2020; Zarocostas 2020). However, a content analysis of social media posts found that the dissemination of misinformation regarding health was more prevalent online prior to COVID-19 (Broniatowski et al. 2022). For instance, a review of misinformation on social media platforms reported that frequently misinformed health topics shared online related to drug or smoking products, eating disorders, and (non-COVID-related) vaccines (Suarez-Lledo and Alvarez-Galvez 2021).

Although youth sometimes struggle to distinguish between credible information and misinformation, they are aware the latter exists, and more than half of adolescents in 2020 (55%) were confident in their ability to recognize misinformation, up from 44% in 2017 (Robb 2017, 2020). Information they frequently seek out in online spaces has included news related to their health and development. They leveraged the power of the digital era and the ubiquitous influence of social media to heighten their knowledge of COVID-19 (Htay et al. 2022), HIV transmission prevention (Young and Rice 2011), nutrition (Skinner et al. 2003), mental health (Carew et al. 2014), sexual health (Mitchell et al. 2014), and gender identity (Pullen Sansfaçon et al. 2020). Some find social media a safe "space" for seeking information. Historically marginalized groups have reported on the benefits of keeping their identity anonymous while accessing online health information—information that would otherwise be challenging or impossible to receive due to social ostracization or stigma (Harper et al. 2009; Mitchell et al. 2014). Pointing to the importance of using social media to disseminate health information, previous research has called for a larger presence of medical professionals in online settings to help mitigate against misinformation and disinformation (Skinner et al. 2003; Swire-Thompson and Lazer 2020).

In light of the U.S. Supreme Court's termination of the constitutional right to abortion and the progression of anti-trans bills in various states, it is imperative to raise awareness of how misinformation in online spaces may be a threat to marginalized youth who rely on these spaces for building a community or for accessing physical and mental health knowledge that is otherwise unavailable to them (Doan et al. 2022; Selkie et al. 2020).

Information Consumption and Mental Health

It is well understood that the consumption of misinformation can influence human behavior; however, little research has focused on how the mental health of adolescents and young adults is impacted. What research is available suggests that a bidirectional or mutually reinforcing relationship exists between anxiety and the spread of misinformation and, additionally, that exposure to falsehoods has resulted in increased levels of stress (Borah et al. 2021; Ecker et al. 2022; Pan et al. 2021). A review of the potential drivers of unintentional (vs. deliberate) sharing of misinformation online concluded that social (e.g., community members, political leaders) and emotional (e.g., anxiety, happiness, sadness) factors strongly influence the likelihood of individuals sharing inaccurate information (Ecker et al. 2022).

In addition to using social media to socialize with peers, youth rely on social media to access information regarding public health (Wartella et al. 2016), which may be not only for convenience or a way to seek information anonymously (Pretorius et al. 2019) but also a means of accessing content that may be traditionally behind a paywall, such as scientific journals and news sources (Middaugh et al. 2022). On the other hand, navigating the sheer abundance of information available online may itself be a source of discomfort or anxiety for youth. Adolescents and young adults surveyed have reported increased feelings of anxiety or stress associated with the consumption of misinformation on social media (Borah et al. 2021; Drouin et al. 2020; Ogweno et al. 2021). Anxiety also is a potential driver of unintentional spread of misinformation. Interviews with young adults disclosed how feelings of anxiety prompted the sharing of emotionally charged misinformation that they mistakenly perceived could benefit the health of loved ones (Hadlington et al. 2022). Given the importance and relevance of information that could impact the health of others, and as a response to their anxious feelings, young adults distributed the information without questioning the credibility of the source. Furthermore, interviewees expressed assumptions that misinformation is less present on platforms where media is formatted differently from Facebook, such as on Instagram, Snapchat, or YouTube. Research has found that these mistaken beliefs may cause youth not to distinguish misinformation from credible information and may explain their motivations for sharing online and for choosing the sources they consume (Hadlington et al. 2022; Herrero-Diz et al. 2020).

Another area in which misinformation and mental health intersect is through cyberbullying and online harassment. Social aggression is prevalent in online spaces, and its negative impacts include psychological distress, decreased life satisfaction, and lower self-esteem, which can particularly impact young people who are seeking social connections (Giumetti and Kowalski 2022). Therefore, it is critical to bring to light how youth have leveraged the online spread of intentionally misleading information (i.e., disinformation) as a means of cyberbullying their peers. For example, teenage respondents shared that they have engaged in behaviors such as spreading inaccurate news about peers, posting hate speech, and creating fake impersonating on-line accounts purposefully in order to harass others online (Maftei et al. 2022). The negative impacts of these cyberbullying behaviors on the targets may include decreased social well-being, self-esteem, and quality of adolescent friendships (Fatima and Siddiqui 2022).

Online harassment and hate speech have also negatively impacted the mental health of specific populations of youth, for example, Latiné adolescents exposed to disinformation regarding undocumented people in the United States while navigating their social media feeds (López Hernández 2022). In response to encountering such disinformation that enforces stereotypes and targets marginalized groups, these adolescents reported having feelings of exclusion and hostility. Another example of the impact of disinformation about marginalized groups was seen following the public remarks about "the Chinese virus" by former President Trump. Gover et al. (2020) postulated that institutional-level displays of stigma or racism contribute to social exclusion and hostility toward marginalized groups. In our research, Asian youth participants have also shared their experiences and aversion toward social media posts that spread hateful content.

> I'm Asian and a lot of my other friends are, so I would usually share because I personally feel that, like, it isn't cool that Asian Americans or Asians in general are being attacked because of something that is outside of their control.
> —*anonymous (U.S.), age 15–17*
> (Smith and Middaugh 2022)

More generally, research has shown that disinformation spread in online spaces may result in increased feelings of social exclusion, hostility, or stigma among targeted youth. Comorbidities associated with online harassment among youth have included suicidality, depression, anxiety, insomnia, and substance use (Aboujaoude et al. 2015).

Who Are Youth Listening To?

Destigmatizing Mental Health Information-Seeking by Sharing Personal Experiences

To understand the relationship between social media and misinformation regarding mental health, it is helpful to have context on how youth typically obtain information. Due to the potential stigma of seeking mental health assistance, many young people find the internet to be an attractive option because it affords anonymity (Pretorius et al. 2019). In one national survey of 14- to 22-year-olds, fully 90% of participants experiencing severe depression had engaged in online research regarding their symptoms (Rideout and Fox 2018). A series of focus groups with Scottish youth found online sources to be attractive to youth as a means of providing access to the personal experiences of others with health problems (Fergie et al. 2013). In line with this, Rideout and Fox (2018) found that 75% of participants with major depressive symptoms turned to podcasts, videos, and blogs to access stories of others with similar experiences. This exposure can lead to destigmatizing the seeking of mental health support and to greater recognition of symptoms and of the need to seek help, as was the case for the 25% of study participants who reported that social media was useful for connecting with support and advice when experiencing depression and anxiety.

At the same time, sharing personal experiences through user-generated content can also be a source of misinformation or can discourage the use of mental health resources. There has been an increase in TikTok users sharing experiences of symptoms of ADHD that are not correctly associated with an ADHD diagnosis (Yeung et al. 2022). In addition, news stories about social media posts that warned against using the new 9-8-8 Suicide Lifeline, which went viral across social media, raised questions regarding how representative the shared personal experiences were among people using the 9-8-8 system and whether such warnings would discourage youth from getting help (Pattani 2022).

How Celebrities and Influencers Shape Information Access

As social media use has become nearly ubiquitous, with 95% of adolescents using at least one platform (Vogels et al. 2022), we have seen a concurrent trend toward reliance on social media for news and information. In a 2020 national survey of youth ages 13–18 years, 77% said they received news and headlines via social media and 39% from celebrities and influencers; 28% reported that celebrities and influencers were their preferred news sources (Robb 2020). In a conceptual review of the factors that influence the spread of misinformation in the health and beauty industry, de Regt et al. (2020) called attention to the ways in which celebrity influencers' promotion of sponsored content has contributed to the spread of misinformation. For example, celebrity endorsements of weight loss treatments, such as Kim Kardashian's sponsored promotion of appetite-suppressing lollipops in 2018, have been identified as promoting harmful health behavior and spreading misinformation (BBC News 2018).

In contrast, Lookadoo et al. (2022) found a beneficial effect of celebrity influencers' impact on normalizing social distancing practices through social media during the early stages of the COVID-19 pandemic. In relation to mental health, researchers have postulated that personal disclosures by high-profile celebrities and athletes such as Selena Gomez, Simone Biles, and Dwayne "The Rock" Johnson can play an important role in destigmatizing mental health problems (Gronholm and Thornicroft 2022) and have been found to be associated with information-seeking behavior (Francis 2018; Lee 2019). As with the tendency to access information from users with personal experience described earlier (see "Destigmatizing Mental Health Information-Seeking by Sharing Personal Experiences"), the celebrity influence on the information ecosystem for mental health can play a useful role in destigmatizing the seeking of mental health information, especially in communities where mental health is not widely discussed. At the same time, uncritical reliance on celebrities as news sources, especially for sponsored content, can be a powerful source of misinformation. Although the practice of celebrities partnering with or referring users to organizations with expertise has been well established in broadcast and print media, celebrity information practices on social media are variable, and norms are evolving.

Algorithms

Algorithms are unique across social media platforms and contribute to the tailoring of the user experience as a means to mitigate information overload, in addition to other purposes, such as recommending and targeting information and increasing user engagement (Qian et al. 2014). Factors that can shape a personalized content experience include personal interest, interpersonal influence (i.e., the influences of online networks as well as offline social circles), and interpersonal interest similarity (i.e., how much online networks and personal interests overlap). Although the algorithms for the personalized experience vary from platform to platform, it has been proposed that platforms' algorithms in general are associated with the type of mental health resources that youth engage with. A critique of Facebook discussed how youth seeking information about health and body image found the platform's algorithm to be harmful, and their mental health was ultimately impacted following their exposure to misinformation about anorexia (Herman 2022). Another study's content analysis of information about physical health and weight loss on TikTok found that a quarter of videos recommended by the TikTok algorithm contained misinformation about nutrition and detoxing (Kilroy 2022). Given that TikTok's largest audience consists of youth younger than 18 years and that more than half of American youth report daily interaction on the platform (Vogels et al. 2022), health professionals working with youth should gain a deeper understanding of digital media literacy levels and how youth navigate social media when seeking information in order to consider its influence on their health.

> The headlines that I see on my social media feed tend to be very sensationalized. This could be due to the fact that social media algorithms promote content which is likely to incite a reaction [e.g., commenting, resharing, or staying on one post for multiple minutes] from users. So, social media algorithms might favor sensationalized news content that is more likely to polarize users. I try to keep this theory in mind as I navigate the news on social media so that my emotional well-being is not as affected by the bold claims I encounter.
>
> *—Sonia, age 17*

Why Are Youth Susceptible to Mis- and Disinformation? How Can Education Help?

Although misinformation and disinformation are challenges across the life span, developmental research provides insight into factors that may be particularly relevant for adolescents and emerging adults. Adolescence is well understood to be a period of rapid growth and reorganization within the brain, creating a window of opportunity to reinforce and build on new capacities while at the same time introducing some temporary vulnerabilities (Selemon 2013). Research in cognitive development has found substantial improvements in the ability of young people to engage in multidimensional analysis of social information (Kuhn 2009), which would indicate an enhanced capacity for analysis of information in social media. However, a temporary period of heightened sensitivity to rewards and emotional feedback during this developmental phase can make it challenging for youth to apply the reasoning for which they have this capacity (Dwyer et al. 2014). Empirical research on adolescent responses to online media found that social factors such as the number of likes or the perceived riskiness of certain content activated the reward response and reduced young participants' application of cognitive control mechanisms (Sherman et al. 2016). These findings indicate the importance of providing youth with opportunities to practice applying critical thinking about media in realistic situations that represent how they might encounter health and mental health information online.

Digital Media Literacy Education

In light of the challenges of misinformation in online media, media literacy education that directly addresses the particular challenges of social media has received increasing attention. *Media literacy* is defined as the ability to access, analyze, evaluate, create, and act using all forms of communication (Middaugh et al. 2022). Many educational approaches to media literacy focus on analysis and evaluation. A meta-analysis of the impact of education of this type, in which youth are encouraged to analyze messages for accuracy as well as for the source's motivation, found a small to moderate impact on media literacy skills and a smaller impact on health attitudes and behavioral intentions (in relation to risky behaviors) (Vahedi et al. 2018).

Research that focuses on youth's capacity to evaluate *online* information, specifically, has found that even when taught media literacy strategies, youth often struggle to apply these strategies in the context of social media (McGrew et al. 2018). One of the challenges of social media is that messages are often presented divorced from the original context, in the form of clipped media that has been shared across sources, often with commentary, and typically in a feed that mixes health information, news, entertainment, and friend and family updates all in one place. The lack of original context and of access to indicators of credibility typically found in editorial news sources and journal articles suggests the importance of media literacy education that considers the unique context of social media. A 2020 survey of U.S. teenagers found that, although exposure to media literacy education is fairly common (with 69% of teens ages 13–18 years learning to differentiate between opinion and news), the kinds of instruction that might be specific to the online space, such as identifying fake news or sponsored content, were far less common (39% and 34%, respectively) (Robb 2020). Middaugh et al. (2022) shared how youth have relied on revocable social media characteristics, such as verification check marks, as a signal of credibility.

> But I really do trust this page. I don't think I've ever gotten something from here and been told that it's not true. So, for social media, it's pretty valid. And I mean, it's confirmed, it has that valid check mark? So I trust it?
>
> —*anonymous, age 19, United States*

Additionally, research on media literacy education in relation to risky content has suggested that it is important to present these ideas alongside engagement with the specific type of content (e.g., exposure to drug use, eating disorder content, or topic-specific news), not just on social media in general. More research is needed that specifically examines what kinds of media literacy education considerations are relevant in the context of seeking and evaluating information related to mental health.

Evolving Technology

Educators and developmental psychologists have sought solutions to keep up with the emerging communication technologies, including generative artificial intelligence (AI) chatbots, in internet searches that youth encounter (Hosseini et al. 2023; Odgers and Jensen 2020; Shurygin et al. 2022). Research has acknowledged the importance of reevaluating data collection tools used with youth in developmental research and theories in social sciences used for training researchers in order to accurately capture the development and experiences of youth in a rapidly evolving digital age (Jimenez et al. 2016; Odgers and Jensen 2020). The gap presented by the rapid emergence of new technologies has only accentuated our lack of understanding about the types of programs or support systems youth may need to navigate digital information in healthier ways (Odgers and Jensen 2020). In light of the infodemic, technology companies have experimented with incorporating new software to detect and reduce misinformation across social media (Kulkarni et al. 2021; Rubinelli et al. 2022). However, these mitigation efforts have met with challenges related to the constant changes in the platforms that individuals use and the complexity of platforms across which they interact (de Oliveira et al. 2021). Therefore, researchers have encouraged the development of programs that support public education about distinguishing between legitimate and false information—even though such initiatives are ultimately left to the authority of unregulated and privately owned social media platforms (de Oliveira et al. 2021; Middaugh 2019). Previous research (Middaugh et al. 2022) has pointed out how youth have expressed concern about the credibility of information on social media when considering the political position of privately owned sources.

> I'd probably scroll past because it's the House of Republicans account, specifically the house of the Grand Old Party account, so I would not really look at it because I don't really side with the Republicans. I also think that, in general,

Republicans haven't always shared the truest information
regarding COVID.

—anonymous, age 20, United States

Furthermore, McGrew et al.'s (2018) study of online civic reasoning in a sample of more than 200 high school students found that 70% chose sponsored content as reliable information, even when it was labeled as an advertisement. In light of this concern, it is important to work toward building dynamic models that protect the vulnerability of users seeking information on social media.

Evolving Users and Their Use of Media

Another challenge in updating educational models and interventions for young people is the general differences in media consumption by age group. A recent national U.S. survey found that television remains the most popular news source for adults older than 50, whereas digital devices are more commonly used by those ages 18–49 (Shearer 2021). An arguably more important difference is in how people use digital devices to obtain news, with those age 30 and older having reported relying on news websites or applications (apps)—which still provide news in an organized format with editorial oversight—compared with those younger than 30, who reported relying on social media. This aligns with research that has found a growing tendency for consumers to rely on incidental exposure to news via social media networks and trending information (Lee et al. 2022) and to prefer noninstitutional sources in social media feeds (Middaugh et al. 2022). The generational differences in how people use media can contribute to a lack of preparation for or resilience to misinformation around mental health among youth, if the adults who make decisions around digital literacy policy, curriculum, or programming for youth have little direct experience with the tools, practices, and patterns of young people's information consumption.

Cultural and Governance Factors

Restricted access to credible information and diverse sources may also be a contributor to youth's susceptibility to misinformation and disinformation. From a global perspective, access to social media platforms varies across governments and countries. For instance, Pakistan, Philippines, Nigeria, and Myanmar offer Facebook to citizens as a free service for accessing the internet, an initiative that has resulted in governmental monopolization of control over what social and health information gets disseminated (Vaidhyanathan 2018). These conditions have led to a proliferation of misinformation and the deliberate misleading of under-resourced, marginalized communities (Nothias 2020). Interestingly, although students in the Philippines reported that Facebook, not a health professional, was their primary source of information, few students actually believe that Facebook is a credible source (Superio et al. 2021). However, the same study determined that students who did rely on Facebook as a source of information also reported higher levels of depression and anxiety. Superio et al. (2021) suggested that misinformation shared on Facebook may negatively influence the mental health of youth and further implored governments to promote programs aimed at reducing the fear students experience when they are seeking health-related information online.

Similar confusion and uncertainty concerning health information and restricted access has been experienced by youth in Western countries (Manduley et al. 2018). In the United States, Canada, northern Europe (i.e., Netherlands and Sweden), and the United Kingdom, youth have sought mental health services or information online due to barriers related to cost and anonymity (Gowen 2013; Pretorius et al. 2019; Scott et al. 2022). Although they are aware of misinformation in online spaces, when struggling to distinguish between credible and unreliable sources, youth often still resort to the latter because credible information is not otherwise available to them. Swedish teens have disclosed to mental health professionals that influencer content containing mental health misinformation has a large impact on how they self-diagnose prior to seeking expert care (Beckman and Hellström 2021). Some suggestions for improving young people's access to accurate health information have included promoting mental health professionals' presence in social media spaces where youth typically seek resources (Gupta and Ariefdjohan 2021).

Promising Practices for Addressing Misinformation

Recognizing the importance of digital media literacy in the context of social media globally, UNESCO (2022) has developed a media and information literacy program to fund and advocate for policies and projects that encourage educators and learners to "think critically and click wisely." One such project is MIL CLICKS, which engages internet users in developing media literacy competencies through peer education in social media contexts (e.g., Facebook, Instagram, TikTok), where they connect with users who want to learn skills to help bring down misinformation (UNESCO 2021). Two important challenges to this kind of approach are that 1) it relies on an intentional community of individuals who are choosing to participate in social networks focused on media literacy and, thus, may or may not reach the everyday user, and 2) learning media literacy practices within authentic social network platforms is helpful due to the differing norms and affordances (e.g., anonymity, moderation) between platforms, but as platforms' popularity or functionality dwindle, the strategies generated by a program that uses currently popular platforms in one era (e.g., Facebook and Twitter) may quickly become obsolete.

In light of the constantly evolving social media landscape, engaging youth as coresearchers and developers of media literacy practices has been identified as another promising approach (Clark and Marchi 2017). Youth participatory action research (YPAR) is a well-established pedagogical model in which adult partners help students engage in critical analysis of local problems, such as mental health services in schools (Kornbluh et al. 2016) and inequitable schooling conditions (Domínguez 2021), and advocate through media for youth-relevant supports and solutions (Clark and Marchi 2017). This approach can integrate media literacy education strategies, such as the use of fact-checking and analysis of sources, but YPAR starts with youth analyzing their current settings (i.e., historical, cultural, socioeconomic, technological), identifying what needs are being unmet for them in those settings, and using the established tools of media literacy education to advocate for meeting those needs.

Conclusion

Although research on the relationship between misinformation in adolescent mental health is still nascent, ample evidence shows that this is an important area for further investigation. Current evidence suggests that social media can play a beneficial role in destigmatizing mental health and creating accessible resources for youth who may not feel comfortable turning to their face-to-face communities. At the same time, the sheer quantity of information, inadequate up-to-date media literacy education, and absence of clear regulation or oversight of mental health information place additional cognitive and social emotional burdens on youth. Thus, it is crucial that we provide young people with the tools they need to take advantage of the benefits of mental health information online while navigating the challenges.

References

Aboujaoude E, Savage M, Starcevic V, et al: Cyberbullying: review of an old problem gone viral. J Adolesc Health 57(1):10–18, 2015 26095405

BBC News: Kim Kardashian called "toxic" for advertising diet lollipop. BBC News, May 16, 2018. Available at: https://www.bbc.com/news/newsbeat-44137700. Accessed February 14, 2023.

Beckman L, Hellström L: Views on adolescents' mental health in Sweden: a qualitative study among different professionals working with adolescents. Int J Environ Res Public Health 18(20):10694, 2021 34682441

Borah P, Irom B, Hsu YC: "It infuriates me": examining young adults' reactions to and recommendations to fight misinformation about COVID-19. J Youth Stud 25:1411–1431, 2021

Broniatowski DA, Kerchner D, Farooq F, et al: Twitter and Facebook posts about COVID-19 are less likely to spread misinformation compared to other health topics. PLoS One 17(1):e0261768, 2022 35020727

Carew C, Kutcher S, Wei Y, et al: Using digital and social media metrics to develop mental health approaches for youth. Adolesc Psychiatry 4(2):116–121, 2014

Clark LS, Marchi R: Young People and the Future of News: Social Media and the Rise of Connective Journalism. New York, Cambridge University Press, 2017

de Oliveira NR, Pisa PS, Lopez MA, et al: Identifying fake news on social networks based on natural language processing: trends and challenges. Information (Basel) 12(1):38, 2021

de Regt A, Montecchi M, Lord Ferguson S: A false image of health: how fake news and pseudo-facts spread in the health and beauty industry. J Prod Brand Manage 29(2):168–179, 2020

Doan AE, Bogen KW, Higgins E, et al: A content analysis of Twitter backlash to Georgia's abortion ban. Sex Reprod Healthc 31:100689, 2022 34933171

Domínguez AD: ¡Venceremos!: challenging school barriers with Latinx youth participatory action research. J Lat Educ 22(3):1208–1222, 2021

Drouin M, McDaniel BT, Pater J, et al: How parents and their children used social media and technology at the beginning of the COVID-19 pandemic and associations with anxiety. Cyberpsychol Behav Soc Netw 23(11):727–736, 2020 32726144

Dwyer DB, Harrison BJ, Yücel M, et al: Large-scale brain network dynamics supporting adolescent cognitive control. J Neurosci 34(42):14096–14107, 2014 25319705

Ecker UK, Lewandowsky S, Cook J, et al: The psychological drivers of misinformation belief and its resistance to correction. Nat Rev Psychol 1:13–29, 2022

Fatima T, Siddiqui MA: A study of bullying on social media among senior secondary school students with reference to gender and type of school. International Journal of Social Science and Human Research 5(2):14096–14107, 2022

Fergie G, Hunt K, Hilton S: What young people want from health-related online resources: a focus group study. J Youth Stud 16(5):579–596, 2013 24748849

Francis DB: Young Black men's information seeking following celebrity depression disclosure: implications for mental health communication. J Health Commun 23(7):687–694, 2018 30111256

Freiling I, Krause NM, Scheufele DA, et al: Believing and sharing misinformation, fact-checks, and accurate information on social media: the role of anxiety during COVID-19. New Media Soc 25(1):141–162, 2023 36620434

Geana MV, Anderson S, Ramaswamy M: COVID-19 vaccine hesitancy among women leaving jails: a qualitative study. Public Health Nurs 38(5):892–896, 2021 33973268

Giumetti GW, Kowalski RM: Cyberbullying via social media and well-being. Curr Opin Psychol 45:101314, 2022 35313180

Gover AR, Harper SB, Langton L: Anti-Asian hate crime during the COVID-19 pandemic: exploring the reproduction of inequality. Am J Crim Justice 45(4):647–667, 2020 32837171

Gowen LK: Online mental health information seeking in young adults with mental health challenges. J Technol Hum Serv 31(2):97–111, 2013

Gronholm PC, Thornicroft G: Impact of celebrity disclosure on mental health-related stigma. Epidemiol Psychiatr Sci 31:e62, 2022 36039976

Gupta R, Ariefdjohan M: Mental illness on Instagram: a mixed method study to characterize public content, sentiments, and trends of antidepressant use. J Ment Health 30(4):518–525, 2021 32325006

Ha L, Andreu Perez L, Ray R: Mapping recent development in scholarship on fake news and misinformation, 2008 to 2017: disciplinary contribution, topics, and impact. Am Behav Sci 65(2):290–315, 2021

Hadlington L, Harkin LJ, Kuss D, et al: Perceptions of fake news, misinformation, and disinformation amid the COVID-19 pandemic: a qualitative exploration. Psychology of Popular Media 12(1):40–49, 2022

Harper GW, Bruce D, Serrano P, et al: The role of the internet in the sexual identity development of gay and bisexual male adolescents, in The Story of Sexual Identity: Narrative Perspectives on the Gay and Lesbian Life Course. Edited by Hammack PL, Cohler BJ. New York, Oxford University Press, 2009, pp 297–326

Herman BD: Meta ethics: how ignoring stakeholder interests endangers Meta/Facebook. Journal of Leadership, Accountability, and Ethics 19(3):58–72, 2022

Herrero-Diz P, Conde-Jiménez J, Reyes de Cózar S: Teens' motivations to spread fake news on WhatsApp. Soc Media Soc 6(3):1–14, 2020

Hosseini M, Rasmussen LM, Resnik DB: Using AI to write scholarly publications. Account Res 25:1–9, 2023 36697395

Htay MNN, Parial LL, Tolabing MC, et al: Digital health literacy, online information-seeking behaviour, and satisfaction of COVID-19 information among the university students of East and South-East Asia. PLoS One 17(4):e0266276, 2022 35417478

Jennings W, Stoker G, Bunting H, et al: Lack of trust, conspiracy beliefs, and social media use predict COVID-19 vaccine hesitancy. Vaccines (Basel) 9(6):593, 2021 34204971

Jimenez TR, Sánchez B, McMahon SD, et al: A vision for the future of community psychology education and training. Am J Community Psychol 58(3–4):339–347, 2016 27726153

Kilroy C: Diets, Detoxes, and Dysmorphia: Health, Wellness, and Misinformation on TikTok (Publ No 172). Master's thesis, University of Nebraska at Omaha,

2022. Available at: https://digitalcommons.unomaha.edu/university_honors_program/172. Accessed November 21, 2023.

Kornbluh M, Neal JW, Ozer EJ: Scaling-up youth-led social justice efforts through an online school-based social network. Am J Community Psychol 57(3-4):266–279, 2016 27215732

Kuhn D: Adolescent thinking, in Handbook of Adolescent Psychology: Individual Bases of Adolescent Development. Edited by Lerner RM, Steinberg L. New York, Wiley, 2009, pp 152–186

Kulkarni P, Karwande S, Keskar R, et al: Fake News Detection Using Machine Learning. Les Ulis, France, EDP Sciences, 2021

Lee SY: The effect of media coverage of celebrities with panic disorder on the health behaviors of the public. Health Commun 34(9):1021–1031, 2019 29565680

Lee S, Nanz A, Heiss R: Platform-dependent effects of incidental exposure to political news on political knowledge and political participation. Comput Human Behav 127:107048, 2022

Lookadoo K, Hubbard C, Nisbett G, et al: We're all in this together: celebrity influencer disclosures about COVID-19. Atl J Commun 30(4):397–418, 2022

López Hernández G: "We understand you hate us": Latinx immigrant-origin adolescents' coping with social exclusion. J Res Adolesc 32(2):533–551, 2022 35470539

Maftei A, Holman AC, Merlici IA: Using fake news as means of cyber-bullying: the link with compulsive internet use and online moral disengagement. Comput Human Behav 127:107032, 2022

Manduley AE, Mertens AE, Plante I, et al: The role of social media in sex education: dispatches from queer, trans, and racialized communities. Feminism and Psychology 28(3):453–454, 2018

McGrew S, Breakstone J, Ortega T, et al: Can students evaluate online sources? Learning from assessments of civic online reasoning. Theor Res Soc Educ 46(2):165–193, 2018

Middaugh E: Teens, social media and fake news, in Unpacking Fake News: An Educator's Guide to Navigating the Media With Students. Edited by Journell W. New York, Teachers College Press, 2019, pp 42–58

Middaugh E, Bell S, Kornbluh M: Think before you share: building a civic media literacy framework for everyday contexts. Inf Learn Sci 123(7/8):421–444, 2022

Mitchell KJ, Ybarra ML, Korchmaros JD, et al: Accessing sexual health information online: use, motivations and consequences for youth with different sexual orientations. Health Educ Res 29(1):147–157, 2014 23861481

Nothias T: Access granted: Facebook's free basics in Africa. Media Cult Soc 42(3):329–348, 2020

Odgers CL, Jensen MR: Annual research review: adolescent mental health in the digital age: facts, fears, and future directions. J Child Psychol Psychiatry 61(3):336–348, 2020 31951670

Ogweno SO, Oduor K, Mutisya R: Sources of information on COVID-19 among the youths and its implications on mental health: a cross-sectional study in Nairobi, Kenya. East Afr Med J 98(1):3390–3400, 2021

Pan W, Liu D, Fang J: An examination of factors contributing to the acceptance of online health misinformation. Front Psychol 12:630268, 2021 33732192

Pattani A: Social media posts warn people not to call 988. Here's what you need to know. Shots: Health News From NPR, August 25, 2022. Available at: https://www.npr.org/sections/health-shots/2022/08/11/1116769071/social-media-posts-warn-people-not-to-call-988-heres-what-you-need-to-know. Accessed November 21, 2023.

Pretorius C, Chambers D, Coyle D: Young people's online help-seeking and mental health difficulties: systematic narrative review. J Med Internet Res 21(11):e13873, 2019 31742562

Pullen Sansfaçon A, Medico D, Suerich-Gulick F, et al: "I knew that I wasn't cis, I knew that, but I didn't know exactly": gender identity development, expression and affirmation in youth who access gender affirming medical care. Int J Transgender Health 21(3):307–320, 2020 34993511

Qian X, Feng H, Zhao G, et al: Personalized recommendation combining user interest and social circle. IEEE Trans Knowl Data Eng 26(7):1763–1777, 2014

Rideout V, Fox S: Digital Health Practices, Social Media Use, and Mental Well-Being Among Teens and Young Adults in the U.S. San Francisco, CA, Hopelab and Well Being Trust, 2018. Available at: https://www.hopelab.org/reports/pdf/a-national-survey-by-hopelab-and-well-being-trust-2018.pdf. Accessed January 10, 2020.

Robb MB: News and America's Kids: How Young People Perceive and Are Impacted by the News. San Francisco, CA, Common Sense Media, 2017. Available at: https://www.commonsensemedia.org/research/news-and-americas-kids-how-young-people-perceive-and-are-impacted-by-the-news. Accessed November 21, 2023.

Robb MB: Teens and the News: The Influencers, Celebrities, and Platforms They Say Matter Most. San Francisco, CA, Common Sense Media, 2020

Rubinelli S, Purnat TD, Wilhelm E, et al: WHO competency framework for health authorities and institutions to manage infodemics: its development and features. Hum Resour Health 20(1):35, 2022 35525924

Scott J, Hockey S, Ospina-Pinillos L, et al: Research to clinical practice: youth seeking mental health information online and its impact on the first steps in the patient journey. Acta Psychiatr Scand 145(3):301–314, 2022 34923619

Selemon LD: A role for synaptic plasticity in the adolescent development of executive function. Transl Psychiatry 3(3):e238–e238, 2013 23462989

Selkie E, Adkins V, Masters E, et al: Transgender adolescents' uses of social media for social support. J Adolesc Health 66(3):275–280, 2020 31690534

Shearer E: More than eight-in-ten Americans get news from digital devices. Pew Research Center, January 12, 2021. Available at: https://www.pewresearch.org/fact-tank/2021/01/12/more-than-eight-in-ten-americans-get-news-from-digital-devices. Accessed November 21, 2023.

Sherman LE, Payton AA, Hernandez LM, et al: The power of the like in adolescence: effects of peer influence on neural and behavioral responses to social media. Psychol Sci 27(7):1027–1035, 2016 27247125

Shurygin V, Ryskaliyeva R, Dolzhich E, et al: Transformation of teacher training in a rapidly evolving digital environment. Educ Inf Technol 27(3):3361–3380, 2022

Skinner H, Biscope S, Poland B, et al: How adolescents use technology for health information: implications for health professionals from focus group studies. J Med Internet Res 5(4):e32, 2003 14713660

Smith K, Middaugh E: Examining social media as a context for positive youth development during COVID. Presentation to the 36th Annual CSU Student Research Competition Finals, San Francisco, CA, April 29–30, 2022

Suarez-Lledo V, Alvarez-Galvez J: Prevalence of health misinformation on social media: systematic review. J Med Internet Res 23(1):e17187, 2021 33470931

Superio DL, Anderson KL, Oducado RMF, et al: The information-seeking behavior and levels of knowledge, precaution, and fear of college students in Iloilo, Philippines amidst the COVID-19 pandemic. Int J Disaster Risk Reduct 62:102414, 2021 34189029

Swire-Thompson B, Lazer D: Public health and online misinformation: challenges and recommendations. Annu Rev Public Health 41:433–451, 2020 31874069

Teplinsky E, Ponce SB, Drake EK, et al: Online medical misinformation in cancer: distinguishing fact from fiction. JCO Oncol Pract 18(8):584–589, 2022 35357887

UNESCO: MIL Clicks Social Media Initiative: MIL Peer-Education in Digital Spaces. Paris, UNESCO, 2021. Available at: https://www.unesco.org/en/media-information-literacy/mil-clicks. Accessed February 1, 2023.

UNESCO: Media and information literacy, in Media Pluralism and Diversity. Paris, UNESCO, 2022. Available at: https://en.unesco.org/themes/media-pluralism-and-diversity/media-information-literacy. Accessed February 1, 2023.

Vahedi Z, Sibalis A, Sutherland JE: Are media literacy interventions effective at changing attitudes and intentions towards risky health behaviors in adolescents? A meta-analytic review. J Adolesc 67:140–152, 2018 29957493

Vaidhyanathan S: Antisocial Media: How Facebook Disconnects Us and Undermines Democracy. New York, Oxford University Press, 2018

Vogels EA, Gelles-Watnick R, Massarat N: Teens, social media and technology 2022. Pew Research Center, August 10, 2022. Available at: https://www.pewresearch.org/internet/2022/08/10/teens-social-media-and-technology-2022. Accessed November 21, 2023.

Vosoughi S, Roy D, Aral S: The spread of true and false news online. Science 359(6380):1146–1151, 2018 29590045

Wartella E, Rideout V, Montague H, et al: Teens, health, and technology: a national survey. Media Commun 4(3):13–23, 2016

World Health Organization: Novel Coronavirus (2019-nCoV): Situation Report–11. Geneva, World Health Organization, 2020. Available at: https://www.who.int/docs/default-source/coronaviruse/situation-reports/20200131-sitrep-11-ncov.pdf. Accessed November 21, 2023.

Yeung A, Ng E, Abi-Jaoude E: TikTok and attention-deficit/hyperactivity disorder: a cross-sectional study of social media content quality. Can J Psychiatry 67(12):899–906, 2022 35196157

Young SD, Rice E: Online social networking technologies, HIV knowledge, and sexual risk and testing behaviors among homeless youth. AIDS Behav 15(2):253–260, 2011 20848305

Zarocostas J: How to fight an infodemic. Lancet 395(10225):676, 2020 32113495

5

Gaming, Identity Construction, and Social Connection

Rachel Kowert, Ph.D.
Kelly Boudreau, Ph.D.
Jessica Stone, Ph.D.

In this chapter we explore the unique networked social spaces that are online games, or video games. We begin with a discussion of games as social networks and how integration of social interaction within a playful shared space has led to co-creative spaces of social engagement (Taylor 2022). This is followed by a discussion of how these spaces are unique because they afford identity production and social connectedness in a different way than what is typically called "social media" or "online social networks." We conclude by presenting a series of case studies that illustrate how the social aspect of gaming can be leveraged for therapeutic intervention, specifically around themes of identity production, sociality, and belonging.

According to the latest market research, well over 3 billion people actively play video games worldwide (Statista 2022). In the United States, more than three in four children (76%) younger than 18 are video game players (Entertainment Software Association 2022). Although video gaming is often considered a solitary activity, video gamers are becoming ever more connected through the ubiquity of networked games. The most recent data from the Entertainment Software Association (2022) support this contention, showing that 78% of players say games provide the opportunity to make new friends; 54% report that, through video gaming, they have met people they would not have otherwise met; and 53% say video games have helped them stay connected with friends and family. Although online games are not often thought of as social media, they should be, because they are one of the most popular online spaces in which social connections are formed and maintained. They not only serve the same core functions as social media but also share many of the same concerns about their impact, both positive (i.e., reduced loneliness) and negative (i.e., internet gaming disorder).

Socializing Through Online Play

Online games are often stereotyped as antisocial spaces. Not only are the players who play online games presumed to be antisocial and reclusive but the space itself also is thought to foster an atrophy of social abilities (Kowert and Oldmeadow 2012; Kowert et al. 2012). These are the messages and images we are given through media depictions of online game players and have come to be part of the common stereotypes held about online gameplay. However, the stereotype of online gamers and the social components of the stereotype hold little weight in reality. For example, research has found no significant social differences between online game players, offline game players, and nonplayers in terms of their reported number of good friends, perceived social support, or social ability (Kowert et al. 2014). This lack of difference reflects the fact that online games are highly social spaces—social networks of hundreds (and sometimes thousands) of people who are congregating, interacting, and playing together. In fact, the integration of sociality into a playful environment makes online games a unique space in the landscape of social networking.

Like other places on the internet, online games are spaces where friendships and social relationships often develop. Although they were not originally designed for this purpose, the social network element of games has vastly grown since the early 2000s. Today, hundreds—if not thousands—of players simultaneously engage in shared gaming spaces. However, socializing within gaming spaces is uniquely different from that on social media platforms. Unlike other social spaces on the internet, online games are interactive, allowing players to engage with others and create friendships through shared, playful experiences. As co-creative systems of networked engagement (Taylor 2022), games create spaces in which friendships are essentially "emotionally jumpstarted" (Kowert 2015; Yee 2002)—that is, the shared, playful activities co-experienced by players allow strong, close, intimate bonds to develop. Friendship bonds are "jumpstarted" through a series of rapid, trust-building exercises (e.g., defeating a difficult enemy) whereby players quickly learn whether they can trust one another before they have even had the chance to get to know each other. Players can then choose to befriend those who have demonstrated their trustworthiness during play (i.e., helping them defeat the difficult enemy). Engagement in a shared activity with a common goal combined with the "emotional jumpstarting" of relationships create a unique social space unlike others on the internet.

In this way, games allow players to strengthen and maintain friendships in a dynamic, interactive, and multifaceted way. This has been found to lead to bonds that are stronger and more long-lasting than those established in other online spaces that lack the element of play. For example, friendships made online tend to be associated with *bridging* social capital, which are the kinds of social resources associated with loose friendship ties that bridge communities, groups, or organizations. This contrasts with *bonding* social capital, which is associated with close, long-term, and intimate friendships. Although social networking has more strongly been associated with bridging social capital (Ellison et al. 2007), both bridging and bonding social capital have been found to flourish in online gaming spaces (Trepte et al. 2012). Further supporting this notion, research has determined that one's co-players are more than just people who can assist with in-game achievements but rather, in many cases, are close, trusted friends (Williams 2006; Yee 2006). Cole and Griffiths (2007) found that up to 75% of online game players report making "good friends" within their gaming communities and, of these, half report regularly discussing their "offline" issues online, including concerns that they have not yet discussed with their offline friends (Williams et al. 2006), indicating the status of these friendships as valued sources of emotional and social support (Boudreau and Consalvo 2014, 2016). Although there is an assumption that online friends are "online only," the Entertainment Software Association (2022) reported that 43% of players play with "online only" friends, whereas 56% report playing with offline friends, 35% with a spouse/partner, 32% with other family members, 25% with their children, and 7% with their parents.

Although online friendships are often considered "separate" from traditional face-to-face relationships, they share many similarities (which may be unsurprising to some, considering the great deal of overlap indicated in the Entertainment Software Association report data just mentioned). In a foundational paper by Steinkuehler and Williams (2006), online gaming spaces were discussed as the new "third place." *Third places*, first described by Oldenburg (1999), are spaces for informal socialization that have the primary function of providing social capital (Putnam 2000), or social resources and relationships, between those engaging in the space. As spaces that provide an avenue for social interactions and relationships beyond one's workplace, home, or school, online games hold the capacity to function as a new third place for informal sociality. Supporting this idea, engagement in online gaming spaces has been associated with the production of social capital through the creation and maintenance of social relationships (Kaye et al. 2017; Trepte et al. 2012; Williams 2007).

Furthermore, despite being formed online, relationships among online gamers are fluid and do not exist in isolation from offline social relationships. As they engage in what is called "modality switching," players often take their online friends offline and their offline friends online (Domahidi et al. 2014). This is, at least partially, because socializing while gaming can take many forms, such as text-based chat, voice chat, and nonverbal interactions using emoticons and emojis. Players engage across spaces, for example, within the game itself using voice chat or in a chatroom-like interface with text. These interactions can be with a small number of other players (i.e., one-on-one or with a small group of players in a specific region of a game) or a larger number of other players (i.e., all players in a specific game or all active players on an entire game platform). There are also opportunities for players to socialize outside of the specific in-game networks—for example, chatting on platforms such as Discord and in online forums. Both are very popular places where players congregate and can engage with the broader gaming community. Thus, even when players are playing different games or using different platforms, they can remain socially connected with a broader network of other players.

Games as Spaces for Identity Production

The unique social environment of games has created a space that is able to foster social connectedness in ways that differ from "traditional" social media, as well as offline relationships. This can have wide-ranging effects on an individual beyond friendship formation to adolescents' developmentally normative work of identity formation. For example, the ways in which teens create their individual identity can be fostered, even bolstered, through engagement within these spaces.

Foundational Theories of Identity Construction

Before delving into the ways that identity construction may, in part, happen within games, we want to provide some brief background on the foundational theories of identity construction to give readers a general understanding of how people construct, negotiate, and understand their sense of self and identity.

Psychology and psychoanalysis aim to understand the contexts and conditions of individual behavior, personality, emotional development, and overall well-being—for example, Erikson's (1959/1994) work on development spanning the life cycle of an individual, Freud's (1940/1964) work on the human psyche, and Lacan's (1949/1977) work on the mirror stage of identity development that focuses on the imaginary, the symbolic, and the real. Lacan wrote that a dual nature of oneself as both simultaneously "self" and "other" makes up the formation of the core of who we are (i.e., the ego) and develops through the process of identity construction.

From a sociological perspective, identity construction is grounded in social interactions and contexts. In psychological perspectives, identity is seen as an internal process within the psyche through *symbolic interactionism*, as defined in the works of Cooley (1902), Mead (1934), and Goffman (1959). However, the sociological perspective sees identity construction as the result of a process of negotiation through social interaction in a cyclical process of perception, interpretation, and response. Thus, the individual develops their identity in a feedback cycle between the external world and their internal selves. Cooley's "looking-glass self" is like Lacan's "mirror stage," in which the individual assesses interactions through the reflections of others and adjusts their behavior in response, in essence constructing identity through the eyes of the "other" within a social context.

In more contemporary terms, within a social-psychological frame, identity is "the meanings that individuals hold for themselves—what it means to be who they are" (Burke 2003, p. 198). According to Stryker and Burke (2000), there are three primary yet distinct uses of the term *identity*: 1) to refer to "the culture of a people" drawing "no distinction between identity and, for example, ethnicity"; 2) "to refer to common identification with a collective or social category," often referred to as *social identity theory*; and finally 3) to refer to "parts of the self-composed…meanings that persons attach to multiple roles they typically play in highly differentiated contemporary societies" (p. 284). Regardless of perspective, at its core, identity exists simultaneously within the individual's sense of self and within social contexts, and its construction is an ongoing process.

Internet and Identity

The internet has enabled people to connect with others based purely on interest rather than on geographical proximity. Due to the anonymous nature of the early internet, works on identity and digital technology of that period discussed it as a place where people could experiment with their identities (Donath 1999; Turkle 1995). As Turkle (1995) wrote in *Life on the Screen*, "the Internet has become a significant social laboratory for experimenting with the constructions and reconstructions of self that characterize post-modern life. In its virtual reality, we self-fashion and self-create" (p. 180).

As a networked social space, the internet allows people to explore and develop their identities beyond the social contexts of their everyday lives. Through a range of expressive forms, such as descriptive text or an avatar, video games and other digital environments remove the limitations of the user's physical body as an identity tool (Haraway 1991). From this perspective, it could be argued that identity construction in digitally networked social spaces offers users a space to explore their identity more expansively than before, beyond traditional and external notions of self, enabling them to explore identities that may be closer to their inner sense of self. Socially, the individual goes through the same identity construction processes described earlier (see "Foundational Theories of Identity Construction"), and others respond to the person's digitally mediated version of self instead of their physical body. This adds an additional layer to the process (and possibilities) of identity construction.

As the internet and digitally mediated social interactions become more and more integrated into people's daily lives, it is important to understand how digitally mediated social spaces and interactions shape users' identities and sense of belonging within digital communities as well as their offline lives. While identity construction may be more fluid and open online, its cyclical process often remains the same both on- and offline. What changes with the addition of an online aspect is that the person now has more possibilities to explore, create, and recreate various identities in a range of realistic and fantastic environments that expand beyond the physical body.

Video Games, Identity, and Belonging

In the context of video games, the literature often focuses on theories of representation (Malkowski and Russworm 2017) and identification (Klimmt et al. 2009), including how the interplay between the two influences a player's personal identity (Blinka 2008; Gee 2003; Waggoner 2009). Discussing the use of an avatar in video games as a form of "playing at being," Rehak (2003) stated that the avatar, "presented as a human player's double, merges spectatorship and participation in ways that fundamentally transform both activities" (p. 103). This not only enables the player to play with and negotiate their perceptions of self and their internalized concept of identity but also allows them to visually change how they represent themselves without making any tangible changes to their everyday physical selves. It could be argued that even in single-player games, despite the absence of other players with whom they can socialize and interact, players engage in social interaction, in this case between their avatars (which they create to represent themselves) and the characters they create in the play process.

Video gameplay has the potential to facilitate the emergence and development of a wide range of identities. Understanding that different games and contexts promote the potential for social interactions and trying on diverse identities, two of the most common types are *discovered identity* and *projected identity* (Waggoner 2009). Much as individuals discover their identity through experimentation and reflection in offline life, players discover the identity of their player-character through the trial and error of video gameplay and, in doing so, can identify with that character, which in turn has the potential to impact the player's own identity (Klimmt et al. 2010). Projected identity happens when players project their "values and desires onto the virtual character" (Gee 2003, p. 55). This occurs when the player sees "the virtual character as one's own project in the making," which is defined by the player's "aspirations for what [they] want the character to be and become" (p. 55). By projecting their values and aspirations onto the character, players can feel that they have a hand in the development of that character, creating a sense of responsibility—perhaps even accountability—for its actions, which are closely connected to the player's own identity and sense of self. As such, it could be argued that, through video gameplay, as the player engages with characters and contexts on the screen, they internalize and react to those events in the same way individuals develop their identity offline.

Community Within and Beyond the Game

Beyond the game space itself, players socialize with others in online spaces such as message boards, video streaming sites, and voice over internet protocol (VOIP) services. As Eek-Karlsson (2021) explained, "for many boys and girls, adolescence is a time for creating and confirming social alliances. A fundamental endeavor in these processes is to belong to a community (both online and offline) and feel a sense of belonging to this community" (p. 1). For many, these game-related social spaces offer the player a sense of belonging to a group or community that they might otherwise not have access to in their geolocated daily lives. Like organized youth sports, multiplayer games can contribute to a player's social identity—a person's sense of who they are based on the social group they are or perceive themselves to be a part of—as they identify not only with the game characters and play contexts but also with other players who share their experiences and knowledge (Scholtes et al. 2016). Although this connectedness may initially develop through the collective act of gameplay, players are able to take their knowledge of the game and share it with others in broader contexts, both on- and offline, giving them social capital (Korkeila 2023) in social situations that, in turn, contributes further to their sense of belonging.

At their core, video games are a medium that gives players the opportunity not only to consume the content but also to play an active part in its unfolding through gameplay. Players engage in games to which they can relate, whether those games are directly connected to who they are in the moment of gameplay or who they aim to be. As digitally mediated social interactions have become a pervasive part of our social world, video games and the social spaces that surround them (i.e., game-adjacent platforms such as Twitch and Discord) offer young players a space to explore worlds beyond their own, which fundamentally contributes to individual and social identity development. Along with the opportunities for identity development, they can participate in player communities that contribute to a sense of belonging they may not otherwise experience.

Case Studies

Experiences in gaming are multileveled and multidimensional. Interactions with both the game software and the other players will elicit and activate complex dynamics within the user. Three sanitized, amalgamated clinical case studies are provided here to illustrate the three prominent concepts within this chapter: identity production, socialization, and belonging. Integration of these concepts in clinical use of video gaming within therapy is essential. For further information, please consult *Digital Play Therapy,* 2nd Edition (Stone 2022) and *Working With Video Gamers in Therapy* (Bean 2018). Informed consent was obtained and explained both in writing and verbally for each of the patients represented in these sanitized examples.

Case Study 1: Virtual Sandtray[1]

- Key concept: identity production
- Hardware: iPad or iPhone; iOS operating system
- Software: Virtual Sandtray application (app)
- Highlighted feature: customizable people

---

[1]Disclosure: Dr. Stone is cocreator of the Virtual Sandtray.

Sand therapies have existed since the late 1920s. Introduced initially by Dr. Margaret Lowenfeld in 1997, sand therapy was developed as a way for individuals to express their inner worlds through creations that can include verbal or nonverbal complementary elements. In this psychological intervention, the user creates a world that represents emotions, experiences, or imaginings that have meaning to them, and the therapist assesses, understands, or intervenes as therapeutically appropriate. Different miniature items are placed within a tray of sand to create a world. Typically, the user identifies (consciously or subconsciously) a figure to represent themselves. This can be a metaphorical or direct representation. When the user desires a direct representation, it is important to have many options available so that the sense of "this is me" or "this is my [parent, friend]" can feel congruent.

In 2011, the Virtual Sandtray App (VSA) was developed for people for whom, and in geographical places where, the traditional form of sand tray therapy was not possible. The VSA is a digital adaptation of sand tray therapy that includes more than 7,000 three-dimensional models and multiple features to allow for customized world creation as well as representations of people, buildings, trees, animals, and more. To assist with identification and representation, customizable "people," or characters, are available to depict self and others. They are categorized by age brackets (e.g., children, adolescents, adults) and can be customized with different skin tones, hairstyles and colors, clothing, and more. As an example of the importance of representative options, the categories are not separated by sex or gender. The models also include an array of emotions and actions to further convey the emotion and interaction within the tray.

This new version of sand tray therapy builds on the theory that identity and representation can be essential to one's level of immersion in an experience. When a person can use figures representative of themselves and others in a virtual environment, the experience can be impactful not only in the depicted scene but also within the user. Being represented can allow one to feel understood and accepted; representation can lead to feeling seen and not invisible and to a sense of personalization and engagement with the story being depicted. Speaking to both digital natives and less digitally inclined users, we found that the VSA expands on traditional sand therapies in powerful, multidimensional ways.

Michael is a 13-year-old eighth grade student who presented for therapy with his mother, who was concerned about the level of anxiety and depression she noticed he was experiencing. Michael expressed his disdain for therapy as well as for his mother's efforts to assist him with his difficulties. He had received mental health services in the past and did not feel the treatment was productive. An agreement was made to attend six sessions of sand tray therapy and then reevaluate the plan moving forward.

During the fourth session, Michael used the VSA to create a scene depicting his experiences at school. He placed a school, trees, playground equipment, and an assortment of young people into the virtual tray. Michael worked diligently on the self-identified figure, who was dressed in a sundress with long brown hair. Michael's physical appearance did not match the character's, which sparked a spontaneous conversation about a longing to present in public as his VSA character in his virtual school. With VSA, Michael was able to create a representation of a current internal exploration and share verbally what the exploration had been like for him over the previous few months.

Identity, representation, and customization are fundamental components of a patient's ability to connect with a projective depiction of their experience. Michael was able to explore various representational possibilities and to ultimately feel that his character communicated important components of himself. The visual representation allowed Michael to complement his depictions with verbal discussion, which is not necessary but welcome when it occurs.

> You can be anyone you want, and if that doesn't work out, you know it's not the person for you. If you don't feel connected to that way of being, then you can be someone else; you can change it.
> —*anonymous VSA user*, personal communication, August 21, 2022

Case Study 2: Rec Room

- Key concept: Socialization
- Hardware: Mobile device, PC, virtual reality (VR) headset
- Software: Android, iOS, PC, console, and VR download

Calling itself "the social space you play like a video game," *Rec Room* (https://recroom.com/) is a multiplayer, cross-platform game environment in which players can meet up privately or publicly and can create their own space or use predesigned spaces provided in the game. *Rec Room* even offers a "Jr. mode" for younger children, which has been certified as "kidSAFE" by the kidSAFE Seal Program (www.kidsafeseal.com/aboutourprogram.html), a Children's Online Privacy Protection Act Safe Harbor program recognized by the Federal Trade Commission. The game allows for the customization of one's avatar, engagement with others in a number of user-created environments, and use of the Maker's Pen to create one's own space. People can see each other's avatar representations and hear each other through the voice-chat feature.

Being able to transport instantly from room to room, environment to environment, allows one to pursue a desired experience. When the player enters into a public space, they have opportunities to encounter people from different cultures, countries, and age groups. Certainly, this can elicit appropriate concerns, just as online chatrooms can. Therefore, it is important for players and parents or caregivers to have conversations about how one puts themselves out into the world and what one accepts within interactions with others. This is a great conversation either to encourage families to have or to conduct within a family therapy session. Knowledge, guidance, and protections such as refusal skills and knowing when to turn to a trusted adult are imperative when a minor is in an unmonitored social space and encounters communication or behavior that makes them uncomfortable.

Erin presented as a 16-year-old high school student who struggled with social interactions in multiple environments. Profoundly gifted, Erin had difficulties finding like-minded peers or even people who held similar interests. She stated she was seeking ways either to find people to connect with or to learn how to assimilate with people at her school. She had a strong preference for the former but had had difficulty achieving these connections.

Erin noticed the VR headset in the office right away. She asked if it was something that could be used in session because she loved using her older brother's headset. After acclimating to the headset model available in the office, Erin asked to go into *Rec Room*, as she had done previously on her own with a different device. Although at times it is more appropriate to create a private space for the therapist and patient to interact privately, in this case it appeared important to witness how Erin interacted socially in this type of environment in order to identify spaces that represented her interests and to provide guidance within social interactions. The therapist also joined, with a VR headset, so that the two could travel together as avatars in the virtual realm. Voice chat was muted for free in-person discussion between Erin and the therapist and was unmuted so she could practice interactive social skills with other avatars when deemed appropriate.

Initially, Erin found preexisting rooms that had themes or activities that interested her. Ultimately, she decided to create her own room with a "build it and they will come" approach. She was able to find several like-minded friends within the virtual space. Cognizant of the need to protect her personal identifying information, Erin did so and found she immensely enjoyed discussions within her interest topics and those of others. She discovered that some of the people who frequented the room she created were going to attend a conference for gifted teens, which Erin ultimately attended with her parents.

The ability to find and connect with like-minded people is powerful, allowing us to differentiate between experiences of isolation or inclusion, rejection or camaraderie. We can learn about ourselves and others through social interactions, and this cannot always be achieved in one's physical day-to-day environment.

"These spaces helped me realize there are people who would want to be friends with me—realize they would like me unmasked, not behaving the way I've been told: [to] 'act normal,' don't act like yourself—that there are people who would like to be friends with me unmasked," Erin reported. "I like to play in this space where, if I act 'weird,' like, myself, nobody would care. [I] realize[d] that can apply to the real world, too, and I can have friends who will like me as I am, both in the real world and online."

Case Study 3: Don't Starve Together

- Key concept: Belonging
- Hardware: PC, Mac, Nintendo Switch, PlayStation 4, Xbox One; not cross-platform
- Software: *Don't Starve Together* download
- Highlighted feature: Up to eight players working together to survive

Don't Starve Together is a branch of Klei Games' *Don't Starve* gaming franchise (https://klei.com/games/dont-starve-together). Gameplay can occur in a private or public world, depending on the desired configuration. These games can be accessed through multiple platforms, but in order to play together, players must access the game through the same platform. For instance, people who purchased the game through the Steam platform can play together through their computers, and so forth.

The game includes spaces for up to eight people to join together with the goal of survival. Numerous environments, creatures, challenges, surprises, and dangers are encountered, and resources must be harvested to feed the group, build shelters and fences, and create various crafts to assist in the team's survival. Resilience, perseverance, resource scavenging and allocation, task assignment, protection, and learning how to ask for help are all important aspects of this multiplayer online game.

Twelve-year-old Adelynn and her family presented with concerns of discord and difficult communication patterns. Her parents were concerned that she was isolating frequently. Adelynn expressed feelings of rejection and being seen as "less than" her high-achieving sibling. Individual therapy was initially conducted with Adelynn to further understand the complexities of her experiences, followed by several family sessions.

All four of the family members attended family therapy sessions and played *Don't Starve Together*. The therapist also participated. After the initial orientation period, which included chaos and many character resurrections, the family began to organize, assign tasks, and work as a team to ensure survival throughout the sessions. With guidance and role-modeling from the therapist, the family began to identify the strengths of each family member, including Adelynn. She began to recognize that she, too, had important things to contribute to the family. Subsequent parental and individual sessions revealed that experiences within the familial gameplay were generalizing to the interactions within the home. The sense of belonging within the family—having importance within the family dynamics—assisted Adelynn with her sense of self-worth and capabilities within the family and into other portions of her life.

"Knowing I have a place in my family, on our team, is not something that happens very often. Playing *Don't Starve Together* showed me—and them—that I have value here," Adelynn reported.

Using a wide variety of hardware and software within mental health settings, and for one's personal use, can elicit a wide variety of benefits. Identity, social connection, and belonging are but three of the experiences one can have. These three cases illustrate and highlight these concepts, as well as the positive impacts recognized by the participants.

Conclusion

Just like other domains on the social internet, online games are spaces where friendships and social relationships often develop. Although games were developed to be play spaces first and foremost, the social element of these virtual spaces has vastly grown since the start of the twenty-first century. These "co-creative systems of networked engagement" (Taylor 2022) are multilevel and multidimensional experiences that foster social connection, identity production, and belonging. The ability to self-identify and represent oneself through play in a dynamic, ever-changing space allows users to explore and demonstrate aspects of their internal and external experiences, find social connection with others, and experience belonging. Rather than dismissing video gaming as a space for unproductive frivolity at best or harmful anti-social isolation at worst, we urge practitioners to consider this evidence that games are unique social spaces in the online landscape and a resource to be explored for its ability to foster connection with oneself and others.

References

Bean A: Working With Video Gamers in Therapy: A Clinician's Guide. New York, Routledge, 2018

Blinka L: The relationship of players to their avatars in MMORPGs: differences between adolescents, emerging adults and adults. Cyberpsychology (Brno) 2(1):5, 2008

Boudreau K, Consalvo M: Families and social network games. Inf Commun Soc 17(9):1118–1130, 2014

Boudreau K, Consalvo M: The sociality of asynchronous gameplay: social network games, dead-time and family bonding, in Social, Casual and Mobile Games: The Changing Gaming Landscape. Edited by Leaver T, Willson M. New York, Bloomsbury Academic, 2016, pp 77–133

Burke PJ: Relationships among multiple identities, in Advances in Identity Theory and Research. Edited by Burke PJ, Owens TJ, Serpe RT. New York, Kluwer Academic/Plenum Publishers, 2003, pp 195–214

Cole H, Griffiths MD: Social interactions in massively multiplayer online role-playing gamers. Cyberpsychol Behav 10(4):575–583, 2007 17711367

Cooley CH: Human Nature and the Social Order. New York, Scribner, 1902

Domahidi E, Festl R, Quandt T: To dwell among gamers: investigating the relationship between social online game use and gaming-related friendships. Comput Human Behav 35:107–115, 2014

Donath J: Identity and deception in the virtual community, in Communities in Cyberspace. Edited by Smith MA, Pollock P. London, Routledge, 1999, pp 29–59

Eek-Karlsson L: The importance of belonging: a study about positioning processes in youths' online communication. SAGE Open 11(1):1–9, 2021

Ellison NB, Steinfield C, Lampe C: The benefits of Facebook "friends": social capital and college students' use of online social network sites. J Comput Mediat Commun 12(4):1143–1168, 2007

Entertainment Software Association: Essential Facts About the Video Game Industry. Washington, DC, Entertainment Software Association, 2022. Available at: https://www.theesa.com/resource/2022-essential-facts-about-the-video-game-industry. Accessed April 18, 2023.

Erikson E: Identity and the Life Cycle (1959). New York, WW Norton, 1994

Freud S: An outline of psycho-analysis (1940 [1938]), in Standard Edition of the Complete Psychological Works of Sigmund Freud, Vol 23. Translated and edited by Strachey J. London, Hogarth Press, 1964, pp 139–207

Gee JP: What Videogames Have to Teach Us About Learning and Literacy. New York, Palgrave MacMillan, 2003

Goffman E: The Presentation of Self in Everyday Life. Garden City, NY, Doubleday, 1959

Haraway D: Simians, Cyborgs, and Women: The Reinvention of Nature. New York, Routledge, 1991

Kaye L, Kowert R, Quinn S: The role of social identity and online social capital on psychosocial outcomes in MMO players. Comput Human Behav 74:215–223, 2017

Klimmt C, Hefner D, Vorderer P: The video game experience as "true" identification: a theory of enjoyable alterations of players' self-perception. Commun Theory 19(4):351–373, 2009

Klimmt C, Hefner D, Vorderer P, et al: Identification with video game characters as automatic shift of self-perceptions. Media Psychol 13(4):323–338, 2010

Korkeila H: Social capital in video game studies: a scoping review. New Media Soc 25(7):1765–1780, 2023

Kowert R: Video Games and Social Competence. New York, Routledge, 2015

Kowert R, Oldmeadow J: The Stereotype of Online Gamers: New Characterization or Recycled Prototype? Proceedings of DiGRA Nordic 2012 Conference: Local and Global—Games in Culture and Society, Tampere, Finland, 2012. Available at: http://www.digra.org/wp-content/uploads/digital-library/12168.23066.pdf. Accessed November 21, 2023.

Kowert R, Griffiths M, Oldmeadow JA: Geek or chic? Emerging stereotypes of online gamers. Bull Sci Technol Soc 32(6):471–479, 2012

Kowert R, Festl R, Quandt T: Unpopular, overweight, and socially inept: reconsidering the stereotype of online gamers. Cyberpsychol Behav Soc Netw 17(3):141–146, 2014 24053382

Lacan J: Écrits: A Selection (1949). Translated by Fink B. New York, WW Norton, 1977

Lowenfeld M: Understanding Children's Sandplay: Lowenfeld's World Technique. Sussex, UK, Sussex Academic Press, 1997

Malkowski J, Russworm TM (eds): Gaming Representation: Race, Gender, and Sexuality in Video Games. Bloomington, Indiana University Press, 2017

Mead GH: Mind, Self, and Society. Chicago, IL, University of Chicago Press, 1934

Oldenburg R: The Great Good Place: Cafés, Coffee Shops, Community Centers, Beauty Parlors, General Stores, Bars, Hangouts, and How They Get You Through the Day. New York, Marlowe & Company, 1999

Putnam R: Bowling Alone: The Collapse and Revival of the American Community. New York, Simon & Schuster, 2000

Rehak B: Playing at being: psychoanalysis and the avatar, in The Video Game Theory Reader 2. Edited by Perron B, Wolf MJP. New York, Routledge, 2003, pp 103–128

Scholtes V, Van Hout M, Van Koppen L: Can people develop a sense of belonging through playing League of Legends? in Proceedings of the 13th International Conference on Advances in Computer Entertainment Technology. New York, Association for Computing Machinery, 2016, pp 1–6

Statista: Number of Video Gamers Worldwide 2015–2021, With Forecasts Up to 2024. Hamburg, Germany, Statista, 2022. Available at: https://www.statista.com/statistics/748044/number-video-gamers-world. Accessed April 18, 2023.

Steinkuehler C, Williams D: Where everybody knows your (screen) name: online games as "third places." J Comput Mediat Commun 11(4):885–909, 2006

Stone J: Digital Play Therapy: A Clinician's Guide to Comfort and Competence. New York, Routledge, 2022

Stryker S, Burke PJ: The past, present, and future of an identity theory. Social Psychology Quarterly: Special Millennium Issue on the State of Sociological Social Psychology 63(4):284–297, 2000

Taylor TL: Games Matter. Washington, DC, Knight Foundation, 2022. Available at: https://knightfoundation.org/games-matter. Accessed November 21, 2023.

Trepte S, Reinecke L, Juechems K: The social side of gaming: how playing online computer games creates online and offline social support. Comput Human Behav 28(3):832–839, 2012

Turkle S: Life on the Screen: Identity in the Age of the Internet. New York, Touchstone, 1995

Waggoner Z: My Avatar, My Self: Identity in Video Role-Playing Games. Jefferson, NC, MacFarland & Company, 2009

Williams D: Groups and goblins: the social and civic impact of online games. J Broadcast Electron Media 50:651–681, 2006

Williams D: The impact of time online: social capital and cyberbalkanization. Cyberpsychol Behav 10(3):398–406, 2007 17594264

Williams D, Ducheneaut N, Xiong L, et al: From tree house to barracks: the social life of guilds in World of Warcraft. Games Cult 1(4):338–361, 2006

Yee N: Befriending Ogres and Wood-Elves: Understanding Relationship Formation in MMORPGs. nickyee.com, 2002. Available at: http://www.nickyee.com/hub/relationships/home.html. Accessed April 18, 2023

Yee N: The demographics, motivations, and derived experiences of users of massively multi-user online graphical environments. Presence (Camb Mass) 15(3):309–329, 2006

6

Children's Online Privacy

Uses, Abuses, and Rights

Valerie Steeves, J.D., Ph.D.

In this chapter, I argue that a push and pull between innovation and protection since social media's earliest days has shaped the online landscape for youth in ways that have too often worked against their well-being. I start with a quick overview of 20 years of research with children to illustrate how the regulatory environment, which has failed to constrain the commercialization of young people's social spaces, has inadvertently shrunk the benefits of networked connection for young people and set them up for peer conflict and reputational vulnerability. I then contrast the regulatory approach with young people's understanding of privacy to better understand the kinds of conditions young people need in order to navigate the online world in ways that make sense to them. Finally, I suggest that a child rights approach can better help shape the online environment to ensure that young people obtain the privacy they need to thrive.

This push and pull between innovation and protection began early in the legislative debate surrounding privacy related to social media. In the late 1990s, there was a global movement to create informational rights to protect privacy in a networked environment (Bennett and Raab 2006). Children were given a key role in the policy debate that ensued, paradoxically positioned both as digitally savvy innovators who would drive the development of the information economy and as young people in need of protection due to their particular vulnerability to online harms (Steeves 2015). The Children's Online Privacy Protection Act (COPPA) of 1998 is a case in point. As the online economy began to grow, activists became concerned that aggressive marketing practices were exploiting children (Montgomery 1996). In response, the Federal Trade Commission (FTC) was given oversight to ensure that corporations complied with minimum standards, such as posting information about their privacy practices, providing access to personal information collected, and introducing more rigorous consent requirements for the collection of personal information from children younger than specified ages. The FTC has continued to tweak these regulations to deal with emerging problems, such as advertising servers and geolocational services, but corporations have largely been left to self-regulate so that they can continue to innovate and develop new information products (see, e.g., Federal Trade Commission 2012).

When issues arise that impact youth, the policy response has been to implement a form of protective surveillance to shield them from the harms of online life. However, this has often unintentionally created forms of protection that work *against* them. For example, to ensure that data collected from young people would continue to flow to governments and corporations, ostensibly to foster bureaucratic efficiencies and commercial innovation, data protection legislation often requires websites that target younger children to solicit parental consent before collecting, using, and disclosing their personal information. While ostensibly increasing parental oversight and control over the information collected from their children, this requirement does little to prevent the commodification of those children's online interactions. Similarly, commercial educational software frequently incorporates broad surveillance technologies that permit the tracking of student activities both at school and at home, again with the stated goal of keeping children safe via constant scrutiny. However, this tracking undermines the open communication and trust that are necessary to foster learning. Perhaps most importantly, these legislative initiatives often fail to protect the kinds of privacy that have been identified as desirable by youth over more than 20 years of qualitative research.

Privacy Uses and Abuses From the Young Person's Perspective

In the early 2000s, when we first started talking to young people about networked technology, they described the internet as a private space just for them where they could hang out, play, and explore the world away from the watchful gaze of the adults in their lives (Environics Research Group 2001). The sense of privacy they found online was central to their enjoyment, particularly for teenagers who were developmentally disposed to try on different social identities and to form strong peer networks outside the family (Orenstein and Lewis 2021). This privacy enabled young people to innovate, often influencing the development of the technology simply by the weight of their numbers on sites such as MySpace, the most popular social site at the time and one where many actively socialized with friends and strangers.

A few years later, in 2005, more than half of the more than 5,000 young people ages 11–17 we surveyed told us that they continued to use the internet on an average school day to explore their interests and to learn about the world, and almost 60% reported that they had pretended to be someone else online to see how it felt to be older, to interact with older teens, or to flirt (Steeves 2005). However, they were starting to notice that the privacy they needed to meet their developmental goals was beginning to shrink. For example, our qualitative participants told us back then that they knew many parents and schools were using tracking software to see if they were accessing pornography online. They had trouble making sense of these concerns, given the high level of explicit sexual content in the mainstream movies they watched and the music they listened to offline. From their perspective, online pornography was just part of a whole spectrum of such content; if it was a problem, it was a problem offline and online, and it was up to adults to regulate it rather than to monitor young people just because they were on the internet. Our participants argued that, instead of surveillance, what they really needed was content advisories so that they could choose the content they wanted to see rather than be ambushed by it. This would both give them more control over what they saw and help them deal with what they perceived as a lack of trust from adults. For example, many youth worried that if they accidentally clicked a link and ended up on a pornographic site, their presence there would be picked up by surveillance technology, but they would have no way of proving their innocence to the adults who were monitoring them (Steeves 2005).

> I blocked my brother; he's like a little spy for my mother.
> —*youth participant,* Steeves 2012

At the same time, our participants still felt they could evade most adult surveillance by taking proactive steps such as deleting their search histories and having multiple accounts with false names. Although they were also starting to worry about corporate surveillance even then, participants felt they had some mastery over it, often entering false information to see what kinds of advertisements they would be served or what kinds of assumptions companies would make about their physical location. In other words, they actively reconstructed a sense of privacy in order to continue to enjoy the benefits of networked connection (Steeves 2005).

By 2011, these strategies were no longer working for them, and young people found it increasingly difficult to obtain any privacy online. For example, our research participants talked about social media as completely surveillant places where they were "spied on" by just about everyone (Steeves 2012). While they had a certain degree of sympathy for their parents and teachers who had "good intentions," their trust in the platforms themselves was eroding quickly; they described the platform companies as a bunch of "creeps" that were watching them all the time, trying to "trick" or "fool" them into releasing information. In a follow-up national survey of more than 5,000 children ages 11–17 in 2015, 95% told us that marketers should not be allowed even to see what young people post on social media, and 87% felt the same way about the company that owned the social media site.

> [N]ow I'm wondering about the creepy people in the corporation.
>
> —*youth participant,* Steeves 2012

Moreover, the surveillance they experienced was beginning to make it difficult for them to meet their developmental goals. LGBTQ+ youth in particular reported that online resources were important to them because they could often feel isolated in their real-world communities, but surveillance made it harder to reach out for community online because of the fear that they might be outed before they were ready (V. Steeves, J. Bailey, J. Burkell, et al.: "Young People's Policy Preferences," unpublished data, 2019; see also Hanckel et al. 2019).

Surveillance Runs Counter to Help-Seeking

In addition, surveillance was unintentionally making it harder for our participants to talk to adults when they did need help and advice. For example, many told us that they were worried about approaching parents and teachers when they experienced online conflict because they feared adult intervention would mean they would lose control of the outcome and be unable to obtain the resolution they desired. Ironically, the zero-tolerance approach that many adults were taking to cyberbullying also interfered with the participants' strategies for dealing with conflict, from ignoring it (with tactics such as blocking or de-friending the other party, which was almost always successful in ending the harassment) or confronting the person face-to-face (making it much harder to maintain the conflict) to mobilizing friends to counter the attack by flooding their social media page with compliments. Contrary to adult concerns that cyberbullying was worse than offline bullying, participants reported that they found online peer conflict easier to deal with because they could capture it and print it out as proof that adults could then act on (Steeves 2012). Rather than pointing the finger at other youth for the conflict they experienced, young people began to place the blame on the platforms themselves.

From Overexposure to Public Humiliation to Social Comparison

Although social media offers youth the potential to explore various emancipatory identities, it also makes it difficult for them to retain private spaces where they can explore without social consequences (Steeves 2015). Moreover, the collection of users' personal information inserts them into a form of surveillance capitalism that is focused on manipulating their sense of self to make them more amenable to commercial messages (Zuboff 2019). For example, the commercial design of social media in particular meant that the young people we studied were constantly barraged by mainstream stereotypical images and celebrity gossip. Moreover, the "Like" button meant that anyone who failed to publicly conform to the stereotype was set up for judgment, which created intense pressure, especially on young females. The inability of young users to protect their private spaces from the intrusion of commercial interests bent on perpetuating these stereotypes and the lack of tools available to them for controlling access to their social media interactions serve economic interests at the expense of young people's social and emotional well-being.

> [Someone commented] "I understand why you're so self-conscious about your weight. If I looked like you, I would be too." That's horrible.
>
> —*youth participant*, Steeves 2015

One participant illustrated how this felt:

> Like, if a girl puts a picture up without makeup on or something, people could attack her.... Even people she doesn't know could see it.... Some people would call her ugly or something, if you don't wear makeup. Or they'll just attack her for that.... They could attack their appearance, or the way you act or relationships with guys, being with guys.... Like, they could say the way you look in general or like clothes you wear or lack of clothes you wear.
> —*youth participant, age 17,* Steeves 2015

Another participant reflected on her experience in high school and recounted how one friend was "just bash[ed]" by a boy on social media:

> I think it was about how she looks. What she was wearing. She had a very authentic look, and she was never really scared to say what she wants or act in any way that she wants. But, oh man, I think it was mostly about her looks, maybe what she normally wears.... Anyway, it was just bizarre.
> —*female youth participant, age 21,* Steeves 2015

Many of our participants told us about the heavy cost they bore when such comments were directed at them, including feelings of depression and a lack of self-worth when others told them things such as, "Oh, I have you around [in photos on social media] to make me look good because you're bigger than me and you're uglier than me" (Steeves 2015). Even when they were not being judged by their peers, social media content made it much harder for them not to judge themselves. One participant explained:

> [T]here's girls on Facebook.... They'll have, like, 500 likes on some of their pictures and...I'll sit there and, like, notice it at first and be like, this person has to be fake, 'cause they're so pretty and they're so photoshopped...but whenever you see them on Facebook you're like, oh my God, they are so flawless.... I don't know, sometimes, it'll make you feel like

crap. It's like, just again setting in, why can't I look like that? Why can't I be like that? Why don't I have these friends? Why am I not popular? And just drains everybody else.

—female youth participant, age 16, Steeves 2015

She concluded,

I think social media is great at giving girls this fantasy world, but at the same time I think it's also really easy to sort of make them feel really bad about themselves.

—female youth participant, age 16, Steeves 2015

Reputational Risk and Young People's Counterstrategies

Once again, young people explained a loss of control over their images as a privacy violation. As one 20-year-old participant put it, "[If] they're selling your information, like your pictures, that's putting you at risk, that is a violation of privacy." Given the potential for reputational damage in such a quantified and stereotyped environment, the inability to "authorize whether or not they use your photos" and to delete a post so "it should not be traceable ever again" were significant limitations in users' ability to manage their risks of reputational harm, especially because the rules were perceived to give social media corporations unfair access to their personal information (Bailey and Steeves 2017).

I'd feel better if I knew that, when I deleted an account or something, everything's gone, instead of them having my information.

—youth participant, Bailey and Steeves 2017

Like, if it's just like, ah, like, I don't know, like a cat or like a TV screen, then I could share it with everyone.... But if it's like my [friend's face] I won't share it with anyone.

—youth participant, Steeves 2019

The reputational risks associated with photos became so concerning that, by 2017, research participants had developed a number of rules to mitigate the harm. First and foremost, they agreed it was safest never to post photos of faces, because faces can open people up to judgment. Second, if they had to post a photo of faces, they selected group shots taken from a distance, but even then, the shot could only be shared if everyone "looked good" and had expressly given their consent to it being posted. Third, there were certain exceptional cases for posting images, such as when the context provided more certainty that the photo would not attract harsh comments. These included photos of faces in which the person is consuming a brand-name product and photos posted on fan sites. In both cases, the poster could be more certain of a positive reception because the content conformed to the commercial design of the platform.

> Because people will judge you, I think. And, like, I don't know. You just—cuz 800 people would see that ugly photo of you and that would—they would probably judge you and stuff like that I think. Yeah.
> —*youth participant,* Steeves 2019

Although the participants in this study talked about social media as a way to stay connected with friends and family, their social media pages had nothing to do with their personal interests or friendships. Instead, they focused on content that a notional audience of "followers" who were presumed to be watching the site would like to see. To select this content, they carefully read the cues built into the application (app) and sought content that would appeal to "everyone." This, by definition, ruled out their own interests or thoughts, which were universally seen as "random." For example, one girl posted pictures of horses on Instagram, even though she did not like horses at all, because "it made a good Instagram theme." Another posted a photo related to the Harry Potter films not because she was a fan but because "a lot of people are fans of Harry Potter, obviously…so I thought maybe they'd think that was cool and, like, two people added it to their collection, because they're, like, big Harry Potter fans, and they liked it." As one boy explained, he would not post anything he was actually interested in because "anyone can access it" and it "might not be appealing or interesting to everyone." In this environment, the safest way to be "interesting" was to hide one's own preferences and mirror the preferences of the online marketplace.

The Hard Work of Reputation Management

Our research participants were also under a great deal of pressure to avoid potentially embarrassing failures. This was brought home when one 15-year-old explained why he decided not to post a photo of a popular television show. He reasoned that, in spite of the fact that the show was a current hit, people in 5 years' time might change their minds and think the show was bad. He worried that, if this happened, his photo from the past would make him look bad.

It is no surprise, then, that so many of our research participants described social media as a great deal of work (Michaelson and Steeves 2020). Finding the right content and managing concerns about missteps is time-consuming and worrisome (Bailey and Steeves 2017; Steeves 2019). Girls in particular complained about the gendered burden when it comes to online communication: not only do they have to manage their own reputations but they also have to manage the emotional responses of family and friends to the content they post, which can be exhausting over time (Steeves 2015).

What is perhaps less obvious is the fact that the early innovative uses that drew young people to social media—the ability to communicate freely, play with their identities, and explore the adult world—have been effectively shut down because of the costs of the corporate surveillance that shapes their online lives. Although our research participants (in this case, youth ages 11–15 years) continued to feel the need to have an online presence, many had retreated and now largely used social media and other apps passively, as pipes for entertainment, because this reduced the potential for reputational damage. They also often blamed adults for never letting them disconnect, pointing the finger at, for example, parents who insist they carry a phone so they can be contacted at all times, teachers who make them submit all their schoolwork online, and employers who text them schedules. They worry that too much connectivity makes it harder for them to connect with themselves and others and report that disconnecting provides relief and the ability to "think deep thoughts." Disconnecting also provides them with some relief from the peer conflict and (self-)judgment that so often detracts from their sense of well-being (Michaelson and Steeves 2020).

Certainly, many of these trends were amplified by the coronavirus disease 2019 (COVID-19) pandemic. Our latest research suggests that networked connectivity can limit the depth of young people's connections to others, leaving them feeling isolated and sad. As one participant explained, relying solely on apps such as Zoom to communicate makes it more difficult to feel a sense of community: "[The] people who I genuinely enjoy hanging out with, but don't necessarily have a one-on-one connection [with] that is anything more than superficial or fun…those are the kinds of friends that I have lost." She concluded that being able to negotiate the line between public and private with others at the same time and in the same physical space is an important part of social interaction because it facilitates the "small talk" and mutual confidence that make social connection and self-worth easier (Steeves et al. 2022).

Situating Privacy Within a Child Rights Framework

Our research suggests that young people's online lives are complicated, nuanced, and stressful, largely because they are unable to find the privacy they seek in networked spaces. It also suggests that there is a significant gap between the kinds of privacy rights we have enacted and the kinds of rights young people need to thrive online. Regulatory frameworks such as COPPA rely on a model that positions privacy as a form of informational control on the user's part. This assumes that a child can choose not to disclose information if they want to keep it private. Once that information is disclosed, protections such as click-through consent and the right to see and correct the data give the appearance of legitimizing commercial use of users' data (Steeves 2009b).

However, young people do not define privacy in this way. They rely on social interactions with others to negotiate a comfortable boundary between what is public and what is private. In networked spaces, this is often expressed as a form of audience control. For example, when most youth report that social media companies should not be able to see what they post, it is clear they know corporations are collecting their data and using it to nudge them, but they maintain that corporations should not be able to do this because corporations are not the audience for whom they are posting (Steeves 2005, 2019). Similarly, when parents and teachers overstep the boundary and intrude on communications meant for friends, this is experienced as a form of "spying," despite the fact that the information itself is published on a publicly available site (Steeves 2012). Young people are seeking this kind of audience control precisely because its lack makes it more difficult for them to maintain healthy identities and to enter into trusting relationships with others.

By way of illustration, consider this story that was shared by a parent several years ago. She had a teenage daughter who had been to a party at which there had been an incident. The next day, when she asked her daughter to tell her what happened, her daughter refused. After 10 minutes of trying for a response, the mother quipped, "Well, if you won't tell me what happened, I'll go online and read your best friend's blog," where, in fact, the details of the incident had already been published. Her daughter was incensed and replied that this would be a complete invasion of her privacy and that, if her mother did read the blog, she would never trust her again. The mother was completely flummoxed; from her perspective, the blog was on the internet, so it was, by definition, public. This view resonates with the regulatory approach to disclosure: if her daughter's friend did not want anyone to know what had happened at the party, she should not have posted the details on the internet. However, from the daughter's perspective, privacy is something to be respected when other social actors work with her to co-create comfortable lines around social roles. From this perspective, respecting privacy can mean simply not looking, even when information is in plain sight (Steeves 2009a).

Regulatory initiatives grounded in a child rights approach align more closely with children's perspectives and needs. This is the approach behind the California Age-Appropriate Design Code Act (2022) passed in 2022, for example, which seeks to update informational rights to better protect children's well-being (Misakian and Young 2022). This Code is rooted in the United Nations' Convention on the Rights of the Child (UNCRC), which was originally adopted in 1989 (United Nations Committee on the Rights of the Child 1989) and, with 196 country signatories, is the most widely ratified human rights convention in the world. The only country that has not yet become a signatory is the United States. The passage of the new California law adds statutory teeth to children's rights in that state, where many social media platforms are based. Article 16 of the UNCRC states that "no child should be subjected to arbitrary or unlawful interference with his or her privacy." More importantly for our purposes, Article 16 also expressly links the child's right to privacy with their right to be free from attacks on their reputation. This language more fully captures the importance of privacy to young people who are seeking to explore their identities and participate in the online world without fear of reputational damage.

The UNCRC also contains provisions that speak specifically to media, including social media, giving us a way to interrogate the commercial practices challenging young people's online lives. For example, under Article 13, children's right to freedom of expression explicitly includes the "freedom to seek, receive and impart information and ideas of all kinds, regardless of frontiers…through any other media of the child's choice," and Article 17 recognizes the important function performed by the mass media and calls for ensuring that the young person has access to information and material from a diversity of national and international sources, especially those aimed at the promotion of their social, spiritual, and moral well-being and physical and mental health. To accomplish this goal, signatory states are required to "encourage the mass media to disseminate information and material of social and cultural benefit to the child." Both articles acknowledge that children's rights may be restricted by laws that seek to promote "public health or morals" (Article 13) or to protect them from "information and material injurious to [their] well-being" (Article 17), but this protective element is balanced by the UNCRC's equal interest in ensuring that signatory states provide children with opportunities to enjoy their rights (including their right to privacy) and that children are able to participate fully in the social world. Again, this resonates more strongly with children's lived experiences, where protective surveillance that oversteps their boundaries makes it harder for children to attain the agency they need to participate in online life in ways that help them meet their developmental goals.

Most importantly, the UNCRC goes beyond mere informational rights and scrutinizes whether the commercial uses of children's data promote the best interests of the child. In 2021, the UNCRC committee released general comment 25 (GC25; United Nations Committee on the Rights of the Child 2021) to address application of the 35-year-old Convention to the digital environment. The GC25 was informed by a consultation with 709 young people between the ages of 9 and 22 years from 28 countries around the world and provided a fulsome understanding of how commercial exploitation can limit children's right to privacy. Article VI(A)(53) speaks to the need to provide online content that is "independent of commercial or political interests," and Article VI(B)(61) states that

> Given the existence of commercial and political motivations to promote particular world views, States parties should ensure that uses of automated processes of information filtering, profiling, marketing, and decision-making do not supplant, manipulate or interfere with children's ability to form and express their opinions in the digital environment. (United Nations Committee on the Rights of the Child 2021)

Clarity on Children's Privacy Rights Going Forward

Most important is Article VI(E)(75), which expresses the spectrum of children's current privacy needs as well as rights, based on today's technology. It even acknowledges children's right to know about anything being done (by industry or government) that affects their privacy, building on the Convention's Article 12, which upholds minors' right to know and, age appropriately, have a say in decisions concerning them; language that has been boiled down in the vernacular to "nothing about them without them." The article states that

> [A]ny digital surveillance of children, together with any associated automated processing of personal data, should respect the child's right to privacy and should not be conducted routinely, indiscriminately, or without the child's knowledge or, in the case of very young children, that of their parent or caregiver; nor should it take place without the right to object to such surveillance, in commercial settings…and consideration should always be given to the least privacy-intrusive means available to fulfil the desired purpose. (United Nations Committee on the Rights of the Child 2021)

California's Age-Appropriate Design Code Act, based on a model code developed by the Information Commissioner of the United Kingdom and enacted into British law in 2021, is a first step toward acting on this more fulsome understanding of children's privacy rights. The code requires that platforms children are likely to access undertake a privacy impact assessment, set defaults to restrict the flow of data, clearly identify when a child is being tracked, and make it easier for children to exercise their informational rights. Much of this merely tweaks the existing regulatory frameworks in other jurisdictions, such as Canada and the European Union, that rely on a narrow understanding of privacy as data protection and informational control. As argued earlier, this often works against the kinds of privacy that young people are seeking. However, the Code also requires businesses to

> consider the best interests of children when designing, developing, and providing [an] online service, product, or feature…[and, if] a conflict arises between commercial interests and the best interests of children, companies should prioritize the privacy, safety, and well-being of children over commercial interests. (California Age-Appropriate Design Code Act 2022, s. 1798.99.29 [a] and [(b)]

Regardless of how the Code will affect industry's privacy practices, GC25 provides essential guidance for intervention and future policymaking, as well as an important model for future work on children's digital privacy. Young people consistently report that networked communication is a vital tool for them to meet their developmental goals but that the personal and commercial surveillance they experience in networked places significantly undermines the utility of that tool. A child rights approach centers youth's concerns and provides benchmarks to ensure that adults create online environments in which young people can thrive.

With the release of GC25, bringing digital rights to the UNCRC, and with the passage of California's Age-Appropriate Design Code Act, we have the potential to ensure that privacy rights emerge directly from the perspective and needs of young people. One hopes the future will allow for youth to be able to use social media safely, for the purposes they envision, and with their privacy rights upheld.

References

Bailey J, Steeves V: Defamation Law in the Age of the Internet: Young People's Perspectives. Toronto, ON, Canada, Law Commission of Ontario, 2017

Bennett CJ, Raab C: The Governance of Privacy: Policy Instruments in Global Perspective. Cambridge, MA, MIT Press, 2006

California Age-Appropriate Design Code Act, AB-2273, c. 320, 2022

Environics Research Group: Young Canadians in a Wired World: The Students' View. Ottawa, ON, Canada, Media Awareness Network, 2001. Available at: https://mediasmarts.ca/sites/mediasmarts/files/pdfs/publication-report/full/YCWWI-student-view.pdf. Accessed November 27, 2023.

Federal Trade Commission: Protecting Consumer Privacy in an Era of Rapid Change. Washington, DC, Federal Trade Commission, 2012

Hanckel B, Vivienne S, Byron P, et al: "That's not necessarily for them": LGBTIQ+ young people, social media platform affordances and identity curation. Media Cult Soc 41(8):1–18, 2019

Michaelson V, Steeves V: "I'll use it differently now": using dual-systems theory to explore youth engagement with networked technologies. Can J Public Health 111(6):1033–1040, 2020 32642970

Misakian A, Young T: California Enacts the California Age-Appropriate Design Code Act. Washington, DC, Foley and Lardner, LLP, 2022. Available at: https://www.jdsupra.com/legalnews/california-enacts-the-california-age-5700283. Accessed November 27, 2023.

Montgomery K: Web of Deception: Threats to Children From Online Marketing. Washington, DC, Center for Media Education, 1996

Orenstein GA, Lewis L: Erickson's Stages of Psychosocial Development. Treasure Island, FL, StatPearls, 2021

Steeves V: Young Canadians in a Wired World, Phase II: Trends and Recommendations. Ottawa, ON, Canada, Media Awareness Network, 2005

Steeves V: Data protection versus privacy: lessons from Facebook's beacon, in The Contours of Privacy. Edited by Matheson D. Newcastle Upon Tyne, UK, Cambridge Scholars Press, 2009a, pp 183–196

Steeves V: Reclaiming the social value of privacy, in Lessons from the Identity Trail: Anonymity, Privacy, and Identity, in a Networked Society. Edited by Kerr I, Steeves V, Lucock C. New York, Oxford University Press, 2009b, pp 191–208

Steeves V: Young Canadians in a Wired World, Phase III: Talking to Youth and Parents About Life Online. Ottawa, ON, Canada, MediaSmarts, 2012

Steeves V: "Pretty and just a little bit sexy, I guess": publicity, privacy and the pressure to perform "appropriate" femininity on social media, in eGirls, eCitizens: Putting Technology, Theory, and Policy Into Dialogue With Girls' and Young Women's Voices. Edited by Bailey J, Steeves V. Ottawa, ON, Canada, University of Ottawa Press, 2015, pp 153–173

Steeves V: Not so social, not so networked: teens' perspectives of privacy and trust on social media. Keynote address presented at the 10th International Conference on Social Media and Society, Ted Rogers School of Management, Ryerson University, Toronto, ON, Canada, July 20, 2019

Steeves V, Crooks HR, Singh SS, et al: "The hardest part right now is being away from school": youth reflect on the impacts of e-learning (dis)connections during the COVID-19 pandemic. Presented at First International Congress on Democratic Digital Education and Open EdTech, XNet Education, Barcelona, July 12–14, 2022

United Nations Committee on the Rights of the Child: Convention on the Rights of the Child, GAR 44/25, November 20, 1989. Available at: https://www.un.org/en/development/desa/population/migration/generalassembly/docs/globalcompact/A_RES_44_25.pdf. Accessed November 27, 2023.

United Nations Committee on the Rights of the Child: General Comment No. 25 on Children's Rights in Relation to the Digital Environment (CRC/C/GC/25). New York, United Nations, March 2, 2021. Available at: https://www.ohchr.org/en/documents/general-comments-and-recommendations/general-comment-no-25-2021-childrens-rights-relation. Accessed May 1, 2023.

Zuboff S: The Age of Surveillance Capitalism: The Fight for a Human Future at the New Frontier of Power. New York, Hachette Book Group Public Affairs, 2019

7

What Makes Social Media Use Enhancing or Harmful?

Understanding Social Media Use and Youth Well-Being

Angela Y. Lee, M.A.
Lara Schreurs, Ph.D.
Sunny X. Liu, Ph.D.
Jeffrey T. Hancock, Ph.D.

In this chapter, we review the literature on social media use and youth mental health to help parents, practitioners, and public health professionals help adolescents take advantage of social media's benefits while being resilient to its harms. Throughout, we integrate the perspectives of adolescents themselves by including their stories about their own experiences with social media.

Social media is integral to modern adolescence. The average teen spends 8.5 hours using their devices—more than they spend on sleep or school—

We wish to thank Research Foundation Flanders (FWO-Vlaanderen), who funded the academic research stay of Dr. Lara Schreurs at the Department of Communication at Stanford University under Grant V400122N.

every day (Rideout et al. 2022). As one high school student from California expressed, "Social media is like the air we breathe. It's just a part of our everyday lives."

However, many scholars and policymakers are concerned that social media is exacerbating the youth mental health crisis (Haidt 2021; Klobuchar and Lummings 2022). As rates of youth depression, anxiety, and suicidal ideation reach all-time highs (Centers for Disease Control and Prevention 2021) and technology companies are implicated in their rise (Wells et al. 2021), public health organizations such as the American Academy of Pediatrics and the newly established Center of Excellence on Social Media and Mental Well-Being have called for more research into the role of digital technologies in potentially exacerbating, or even causing, mental health issues in adolescents (American Academy of Pediatrics 2021). Empirically informed guidance can support parents and practitioners in helping adolescents engage with social media in healthy, responsible ways.

Scaffolding healthy engagement with social media can be challenging. By providing short-term rewards such as social validation, distraction, and entertainment (Sun and Zhang 2021), social media can undermine youth well-being by displacing other endeavors, such as spending time with family and studying. It can also be difficult for children and adolescents to resist the pull of spending time online (Hall and Liu 2022; Schou Andreassen et al. 2016) or comparing themselves with others (Kleemans et al. 2018). Indeed, seeing curated images of hyper-idealized beauty standards and unattainable lifestyles may harm self-esteem and body image.

Efforts to protect youth from these challenges often involve urging them to reduce their engagement with social media, such as by setting strict limits on screen time or taking devices away. Although well-intentioned, wholesale efforts to reduce social media use can also have negative consequences on adolescent mental health (Radtke et al. 2022). After all, there are many ways in which social media use can provide meaningful, tangible benefits to children and adolescents. Nowhere was this more evident than during the coronavirus disease 2019 (COVID-19) pandemic, which forced schools to close and young people to stay home (Panchal et al. 2023). This time of social isolation was challenging for all, but students with access to digital tools such as social media were less depressed and anxious than their digitally isolated peers because they could better maintain their friendships (Metherell et al. 2022; Minihan et al. 2023). Especially when in-person activities are limited, social media can be an essential source of social connection and emotional support. As one high school student from Texas said, "Having social media was a lifeline during COVID-19. Even though the world was burning down and everything was awful, at least I could still talk to my friends and see funny memes of people still finding ways to make others laugh. [Social media] really helped me feel less alone when I was stuck at home and there was nothing good happening in the world."

Social media can also support well-being during more normal times. For instance, it can help teens maintain valued relationships with their friends even if they no longer live in the same city, go to the same schools, or take part in the same activities (Ellison et al. 2007; Steinfield et al. 2013). Social media sites can also connect teens with new sources of support through affinity groups for specific identities and interests hosted on subReddits (discussion boards for specific topics on Reddit) or sides of TikTok (informal content networks organized around algorithmic personalization) (Katz et al. 2022; Lee et al. 2022). Being able to find and participate in communities of "people like them" can be particularly beneficial for adolescents from marginalized backgrounds, such as LGBTQ+ teens or those who are part of an underrepresented ethnic minority (Cavalcante 2019; Hiebert and Kortes-Miller 2021; Lucero 2017).

What Do We Know About the Effects of Social Media on Well-Being?

To date, hundreds of empirical studies have examined the relationship between social media use and diverse indicators of psychological well-being (Meier and Reinecke 2021; Valkenburg et al. 2022). However, studies find conflicting effects of social media use on various well-being indicators. For instance, whereas some research indicates that social media exacerbates loneliness by displacing time spent with friends in person, other studies find that it mitigates loneliness through connections with people online, while still others find no effects whatsoever (O'Day and Heimberg 2021).

We find similar mixed results when we examine the state of the field overall. Meta-analyses and systematic reviews find inconsistent associations between social media use and mental health (Meier and Reinecke 2021; Valkenburg et al. 2022). In an analysis of 226 studies spanning more than 275,000 participants, Hancock et al. (2022) found small but significant associations between social media use and well-being. For the average person, using social media for longer periods of time is associated with feeling not only slightly more depressed and anxious but also slightly more socially connected and emotionally supported. These small effects align with other work showing that technology has a much weaker, and less harmful, effect on well-being than often purported (Orben and Przybylski 2019). Together, these findings may help allay concerns that social media is as harmful for adolescents' mental health as is often feared (Orben 2020).

Indeed, for the average teen, spending more time on social media does not necessarily worsen their mental health. Beyens et al. (2020) found that spending more time on social media enhanced well-being for 46% of adolescents, undermined well-being for 10%, and had no effect on 44%. Similarly, social media was shown to affect different individuals' self-esteem, depression, anxiety, and stress in different ways (Valkenburg et al. 2022).

What Makes Social Media Use Enhancing or Harmful?

Why is social media enhancing for some adolescents and harmful for others? Understanding these heterogeneous effects requires us to identify the psychological factors that make an adolescent more or less vulnerable to social media influences. In doing so, we need to look beyond screen time (Valkenburg et al. 2022) and consider how adolescents are engaging with social media, how they feel about their activity, and what they are seeing online. Considering diverse elements of social media experiences is important; young people use a variety of social media platforms, in diverse ways, to achieve different kinds of goals—some of which can enhance their mental health, whereas others may undermine it (Bayer et al. 2020).

Content

First, we need to consider what *content* adolescents are seeing and posting on social media. For instance, the effects of social media on self-esteem, body image, and body dysmorphia are closely tied to specific types of content (Meier and Reinecke 2021; Odgers and Jensen 2020). Although seeing photos of nature or art may not undermine an youth's body image, interacting with posts from celebrities and influencers such as Chris Hemsworth or Kylie Jenner that depict unrealistic beauty standards may make the youth feel worse about their own appearance (Kleemans et al. 2018). Given the norms around posting one's "best self" on social media (Schreurs and Vandenbosch 2022), teenagers may also see their own peers sharing perfected images of themselves—either carefully posed and selected from a series of photos (e.g., a "burst") or edited with filters that allow them to brighten their complexion, blur their skin, or even reshape their bodies (e.g., with the Facetune application). Exposure to such content can harm mental health by increasing adolescents' body dissatisfaction (Kleemans et al. 2018).

Beyond physical appearances, seeing idealized content that showcases the "highlights" of others' lives can also undermine well-being by eliciting social comparison. Adolescents may feel sad or envious if they constantly see their peers on vacation, going to parties, or celebrating professional or relational milestones on sites such as Instagram (Chae 2018; Krasnova et al. 2015). One high school student who identified as being low-income said that looking at the feeds of their classmates made them feel insecure about their own upbringing: "I remember when I went to high school and got Instagram and then I was like, whoa. People go on vacation all the time? They get new clothes and look like models all the time?... I felt embarrassed to post much about my own life when I [saw] theirs."

Different adolescents can also interpret the same kind of social media content in different ways. Teens who feel secure in their friendships, for example, may not feel insecure or experience a "fear of missing out" (FOMO) when they see their peers hanging out together. However, this could exacerbate feelings of loneliness for teens who already feel left out. It is important to note that the effects of social media content on mental health interact with the broader *context* of individuals' lives.

Sometimes social media really makes you sad. You don't always know why. But then you don't want to use it anymore. Or when I am going through a bad time. Then I do not want to use social media. I don't want to fake it for everyone. That's the thing, people act on social media like they are super happy but that's not always the case. Then I don't want to be scrolling on social media and see how happy everyone is. In that case I just want to log out; it is too much effort.

—*anonymous female adolescent, Belgium*

Exposure to hurtful, offensive, or hateful comments can also clearly harm adolescents' mental health (Giumetti and Kowalski 2022; Walther 2022). Individuals can be targeted by cyberbullying through private channels (e.g., in Instagram direct messaging and video game chats), public forums (e.g., comments), and social media content designed to mock the victim (e.g., memes). Seeing online aggression that targets communities or identities, such as racist, sexist, or homophobic content, can also harm well-being. A recent review of Black youth's experiences with social media found that it often exposed them to private and public forms of racial discrimination (Park et al. 2024). One Black teen from California described the impact of seeing waves of racist comments attempting to justify or dismiss police brutality during the protests around the murder of George Floyd Jr. as "incredibly depressing," to the point where he needed to take time away from social media altogether.

Motivations

In addition to examining what they are doing and seeing online, it is also important to consider *why* teens engage with certain types of content. They use social media for diverse reasons that range from entertainment and relaxation to learning and building relationships. For example, one teenage female reported watching YouTube videos "every day to go to sleep" because certain kinds of sounds (e.g., autonomous sensory meridian response [ASMR] videos) helped her unwind for the night. Several teenage males described using social media to try to boost their social status, spending afternoons after school making funny or engaging TikTok videos in hopes of going viral and "getting clout." Social media can also be a valuable way for youth to express their opinions and influence others. Two college students described themselves as "BookTok creators," referencing a TikTok subcommunity organized around finding and sharing particular types of books.

These myriad uses of social media can be driven by diverse motivations, which may have important implications for users' well-being. Take, for instance, a high school female who spends 20 minutes looking at her friends' Instagram profiles. Using social media in this way may be beneficial if she is reminiscing about positive memories with her friends. On the other hand, seeing photos of her friends may harm her mental health if driven by anxiety. As one middle school girl said, "Sometimes I check [Instagram] stories, but then I feel bad when I see my friends hanging out without me. Then I have to go look and see what [the other friends] posted. What if they're leaving me out?" In this scenario, this student is spending the same amount of time on social media and looking at the same content. However, the different motivations underlying her social media use can shape whether she feels better or worse (Meier and Reinecke 2021).

The specific affordances of social media platforms can also introduce new motivations for sharing content, with differing effects on youth well-being. Sites such as Instagram and TikTok allow individuals to share content to a wide audience of friends, followers, and strangers on the internet. As a result, teens may use social media pragmatically as a form of social compensation to help them find the social connection and closeness they desire when their face-to-face interactions are unfulfilling or infrequent (Hancock et al. 2022). However, many teens may also be motivated to post content out of a desire to receive positive peer feedback in the form of likes and positive comments (Sabik et al. 2020). Posting for social validation may result in "strategically" deployed content that mainly aims to impress others. Adolescents who care deeply about the likes and followers they get on social media may try to "perform" an idealized version of their lives to maintain a positive self-presentation (Casares and Binkley 2022). Such positively biased self-presentations may, however, undermine adolescents' well-being because they are likely to represent inauthentic reflections of the self (Bailey et al. 2020).

Mindsets

The beliefs teens have about their social media use can also affect their mental health and well-being. For instance, some adolescents describe their social media use as a "powerful tool," something they can use to "connect with [their] friends all the time" and to "try out new ways of expressing [themselves]." Others, however, view social media as an addiction. As one high school student said, "I worry about spending way too much time on social media. I feel like I can open TikTok and just get sucked in for hours. I had to delete my app [application] because I couldn't resist it."

These beliefs can be understood as social media *mindsets*, which are powerful core assumptions about the nature of things in our lives (Lee and Hancock 2020). Just as prior research on education showed that people can have mindsets about their own intelligence (e.g., a growth or fixed mindset) (Dweck 2008; Yeager and Dweck 2012), people understand their social media use in terms of the amount of agency they have over social media (high vs. low) and the expected valence of its effects on their lives (positive vs. negative) (Lee et al. 2021). Youth who believe that their social media use is an addiction could be understood as having a low-agency, negative mindset because they see themselves as having little control over their engagement with a harmful habit. On the other hand, teens who see their social media use as something they can use to pursue meaningful goals—such as social connection—have a high-agency, positive mindset.

High agency and positive mindsets are positively associated with well-being (Lee and Hancock 2020). People who viewed themselves as in control of their social media use reported not only greater life satisfaction and perceived social support but also less depression, anxiety, and stress. In contrast, people with the mindset that they had little control over their social media use experienced more psychological distress.

Mindsets are consequential to well-being because they change how people make sense of the time they spend with social media. For instance, someone who feels that their social media use is out of their control may interpret an hour spent browsing content from friends as a failure to manage their time effectively, with potential negative ramifications for their productivity (Cheng et al. 2019; Lanette et al. 2018). As a result, they may feel disappointed in themselves, resulting in a more depressed mood and a reduced sense of self-efficacy (Du et al. 2019, 2021). In contrast, an individual with a more empowered mindset might view the same period of use as a meaningful opportunity to fulfill important social and relational goals. They may focus on the positive activities they were able to do because of social media, such as building stronger relationships or finding new connections (Dolan et al. 2016; Pelletier et al. 2020). Having a more agentic and positive mindset may therefore help adolescents obtain benefits from their social media use while also maintaining a positive self-image.

Social Media Literacy

Another important determinant of social media effects pertains to social media literacy. *Social media literacy* is "the extent to which cognitive and affective structures are present among users to ensure the risks of interactions with social media content are mitigated and the opportunities are maximized" (Schreurs 2022, p. 21). When adolescents understand the unique ways in which social media works, they can be more resilient to specific threats and obtain greater benefits from their use. For instance, teaching adolescents that social media content is often warped by a positivity bias in which people try to put their "best foot forward" and create a highlight reel of their best moments can help protect adolescents from the risks of being exposed to idealized photos online. In a focus group study, Burnette et al. (2017) found that girls with high levels of social media literacy were less prone to draw harmful comparisons between the idealized images they saw and their own bodies because they could reason about the artificial nature of idealized content and the techniques used to produce these perfected images (e.g., Photoshop applications). One experiment among young adult women also showed that increasing social media literacy reduced the negative impact of exposure to idealized appearance content on social media on body satisfaction (Tamplin et al. 2018).

In our qualitative research, youth also attested to the use of social media literacy skills in their interactions with idealized content. This seemed to manifest itself, for instance, in critical thinking about users' motivations for posting such content as well as a critical understanding of its unrealistic nature, which helps reduce harmful social comparison processes. As one participant in Belgium said, "I also keep in mind that they want to show the most perfect image. They posted it, and it's unfortunate that I saw it, but I also have perfect moments when they are not having a nice time." Another added, "I never compare myself to others on social media. Because when you do that, you would try to attain something which in the end, you will never be able to attain. So why would you do that?"

Contexts

Finally, it is important to consider the *contexts* in which adolescents engage with social media. Their social and family environments also play a significant role in their social media experiences (Masur et al. 2022). Social support and social capital are tangible and intangible assistance and resources that individuals can receive from both their online and offline social networks.

Social media platforms connect people's strong and weak ties, merge their online and offline networks, and expand the sizes of their networks. Yet teens' social media experience and the support and capital they can pull from social media depend on what kinds of resources are available on social media for them and whom they talk with, follow, and are followed by in social media spaces. Sociocultural factors, such as class, race, and culture, determine teens' network and contextual characteristics. These network and contextual features not only influence what types of content they see but also the qualities of interactions and experiences they have on social media. For instance, negative stereotypes of Black people displayed on social media can be internalized by Black adolescents. Such content gives rise to diminished psychological well-being of Black youth (Smith 2020). In addition, teens from upper-class families, compared with the teens from lower-class families, are more likely to have social capital and resources in their network that they can tap into for academic and self-growth support (Livingstone and Blum-Ross 2020).

How Can We Improve Teens' Experiences With Social Media?

Understanding the effects of social media on mental health can help adults support the young people in their lives. As reflected in the literature, social media use is neither universally harmful nor universally helpful. Rather, the way social media use influences adolescent mental health is dependent on several factors, including the content they see, their motivations for using social media, the context of their use, and the mindsets they hold about the role of social media in their lives. What can parents, practitioners, and public health professionals do to support young people in engaging with social media in beneficial ways? Figure 7–1 demonstrates some potential approaches.

"Be Curious, Not Furious": Ask About Uses and Motivations

Adults should have an open mind about children and adolescents' social media use. Social media seems here to stay, and parents and practitioners should find ways to help children and adolescents navigate its affordances and challenges without labeling social media overall as "bad" (Yang et al. 2021). Indeed, conversations with adolescents reveal that many teens believe their parents do not trust them when it comes to their social media use. In an activity in which they reflected on what they wish their parents knew about their technology use, they wrote things such as "I wish my parents would understand that I'm not always on my phone"; "I wish my parents would notice that I don't make bad decisions online"; and "I want my parents to talk to me about what I'm doing online. It's not all bad, and it can actually be really interesting!" The literature on parental mediation theory may offer some valuable insights on how to navigate these conversations. Specifically, we can see several different ways that parents—or any guardian or caretaker—can manage and regulate children's experiences with media (Clark 2011). Essentially, three types of mediation can be distinguished: active mediation, restrictive mediation, and co-use.

Active mediation refers to parents talking with their children about the media they use and explaining things they encounter as part of an ongoing dialogue. *Restrictive mediation* concerns the rules, regulations, and limitations parents impose on their children's media. The third type, *co-use,* means using media together (Clark 2011; Shin and Lwin 2022). Of these, active mediation has most consistently been found to mitigate potential negative effects of media viewing (Clark 2011). Many adults may feel less confident engaging in active mediation strategies in today's rapidly evolving digital world, particularly if they believe that the adolescents in their lives have more expertise in digital media than they do (Van den Bulck et al. 2016). As a result, they may fall back on restrictive mediation strategies more often (Lwin et al. 2021). Nonetheless, when parents do engage in active mediation of adolescents' digital media use, this may have positive consequences. Research has found that active parental mediation can increase adolescents' digital skills (Sánchez-Valle et al. 2017), their social media literacy (Schreurs 2022), and their fundamental beliefs about the values of technology (Liu et al., under review), hinting at the importance of this mediation style to sup-

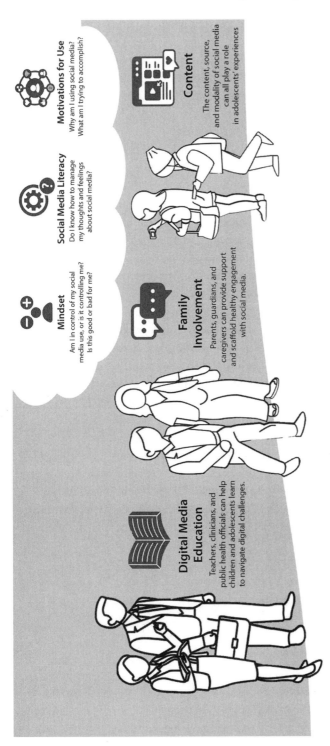

Motivations for Use
Why am I using social media? What am I trying to accomplish?

Social Media Literacy
Do I know how to manage my thoughts and feelings about social media?

Mindset
Am I in control of my social media use, or is it controlling me? Is this good or bad for me?

Content
The content, source, and modality of social media can all play a role in adolescents' experiences

Family Involvement
Parents, guardians, and caregivers can provide support and scaffold healthy engagement with social media.

Digital Media Education
Teachers, clinicians, and public health officials can help children and adolescents learn to navigate digital challenges.

Figure 7–1. Supporting healthy adolescent engagement with social media.

Adolescent social media use is complex and informed by their individual characteristics as well as their support systems. The extent to which using social media is helpful or harmful for their mental health is shaped by the 1) content they are engaging with, 2) their motivations for using social media, 3) their mindset about social media's role in their life, and 4) their literacy about how to process and respond to what they see on social media. Parents and guardians can support healthy youth engagement with social media by having open conversations about the digital part of teens' lives and helping them develop an empowered, agentic mindset toward their use. Finally, teaching teens how best to interact with digital media in their lives through formal or informal education can support them in navigating the potential challenges inherent to digital life.

port the minimization of risks and the maximization of opportunities for their adolescents' social media use.

The research on active parental mediation indicates that parents do not need to be knowledgeable about all types of social media to empower and support their children. Having open conversations about social media experiences and engaging in reasoning-oriented discussion can help adolescents develop the skills needed to mitigate negative and enhance positive social media effects (Schreurs 2022). Parents and adults should try to create a safe space for adolescents to voice their social media concerns and experiences. In doing so, they can display a healthy amount of curiosity while at the same time respecting the independence adolescents need to explore on their own (Lwin et al. 2021; Schreurs 2022; Valkenburg and Piotrowski 2017). To facilitate this type of discussion, parents are advised to stay abreast of their children's social media activities not only by listening to their children's accounts of their experiences but also by consulting resources that guide parents and provide information about current social media trends in this developmental group (Schreurs 2022; Shin and Lwin 2022). Such parental strategies can help adolescents when they independently interact with social media and can thus result in optimal usage patterns.

To this end, practitioners could develop education materials that advance parents' active mediation skills. These materials could introduce ways to start and facilitate discussions about social media in addition to providing tips on how parents could make time for such conversations (Lwin et al. 2021). Practitioners working with adolescents directly are also advised to actively listen to their social media experiences and determine the quality of and the underlying psychological processes characterizing their use, rather than focusing on the amount of time they spend on these platforms (Yang et al. 2021). A climate in which adults close to the adolescent seem genuinely interested in how they use social media, without assuming it is all negative, can make the adolescent more willing to confide in these adults should they encounter distressing content or experience negative interactions (Yang et al. 2021). As such, there may be more opportunities for parents and practitioners to intervene if needed.

Beyond Screen Time Restrictions: Supporting Agentic Social Media Use

In a similar vein, adults should consider supporting young people in *taking control* of their own social media use rather than attempting to restrict it or manage it themselves (Lee and Hancock 2024; Lee et al. 2023). Although it can often be tempting to believe that taking devices away or removing adolescents' access to the internet will be sufficient to protect them from its potential harms (Liao and Sundar 2022), empirical research does not support the efficacy of such approaches (Radtke et al. 2022). Instead, students who are forced to reduce their social media use or to stop using their devices generally spend the time on other media instead, such as television, movies, or video games, or simply end up lying about the time they spend online (Przybylski et al. 2021). More importantly, these "digital detoxes" do not necessarily improve mental health. In fact, removing access to social media can even backfire by cutting off valuable sources of social connection and emotional support, which are particularly important during adolescence.

Adopting a restriction-only approach to managing youth engagement with social media has other consequences as well. Notably, such an approach does not help young people learn to manage and live with their own social media use in the longer term. Research on scaffolding emphasizes the importance of helping children and adolescents learn to regulate themselves (Van der Stuyf 2002), whether this means teaching them how to process and cope with their emotions or how to plan for the future. Taking devices away prevents them from engaging in this valuable process of learning to take control of their social media use and may even set them up for a cycle of forever trying to obtain the "forbidden fruit." One college student remarked that after having their phone constantly taken away from them as punishment when they were an adolescent, they felt more compelled to use it for longer when they went off to school on their own.

Teaching adolescents how to use social media *agentically* is a viable alternative to attempting to reduce their use. This means supporting young people in engaging with social media in ways that emphasize having the beliefs, knowledge, and practices to use it intentionally (Lee and Hancock 2024; Lee et al. 2023). Compared with those who "mindlessly" use social media use, people who use it agentically do so with a purpose in mind: they leverage the affordances of social media to do things that are meaningful, useful, or satisfying for them. This builds on research showing that people who have high-agency mindsets about social media are not only in more control of their social media use but also use it in more intentional ways (Lee and Hancock 2023). We can support young people in using social media agentically by equipping them with the tools they need to take advantage of its positive aspects while being aware and responsive to its digital harms. Rather than taking devices away or setting a predetermined allotment of screen time, parents may instead have a conversation with their children that supports them in reflecting on their social media use and in developing their own boundaries. By asking young people to reflect on "how much is too much?" and how they can recognize when they are beginning to spend too much time on social media, adults can scaffold the development of children's skills in managing their own use.

Treat Social Media as an Opportunity for Teens' Development, Not as a Scapegoat

Parents and health professionals can adopt more nuanced perspectives on social media. Instead of treating it as a type of addictive, harmful, and manipulative technology, we can embrace this technology as an opportunity for adolescents' growth and development. Teens can use social media for learning and skill development. They learn a lot from social media and thus become experts in their interests and hobbies. They can also use social media to practice interpersonal and social skills, such as when it is appropriate to send a friend request to their teachers and how best to communicate with family or other adults in their networks using direct messages. So instead of blaming social media for kids' inadequate interpersonal skills or waste of study time, parents and health professionals can find ways to use social media for their teens' growth.

Conclusion

There is no denying that social media is integral to the lives of today's children and adolescents. However, understanding its effects on their mental health requires considering the ways they use it, the content they see, and their mindset toward technology. Social media is in no way unequivocally negative, and the risks and opportunities that adolescents encounter when using it differ depending on the context of their use. Individual characteristics as well as adolescents' social environment shape their social media use, and parents and guardians can support healthy engagement by having open conversations about social media. Such conversations can help adolescents develop an empowered, agentic mindset that ultimately minimizes the challenges and maximizes the opportunities inherent to digital life.

References

American Academy of Pediatrics: AAP-AACAP-CHA Declaration of a National Emergency in Child and Adolescent Mental Health. Washington, DC, American Academy of Pediatrics, October 19, 2021. Available at: https://www.aap.org/en/advocacy/child-and-adolescent-healthy-mental-development/aap-aacap-cha-declaration-of-a-national-emergency-in-child-and-adolescent-mental-health. Accessed November 29, 2023.

Bailey ER, Matz SC, Youyou W, et al: Authentic self-expression on social media is associated with greater subjective well-being. Nat Commun 11(1):4889, 2020 33024115

Bayer JB, Triệu P, Ellison NB: Social media elements, ecologies, and effects. Annu Rev Psychol 71:471–497, 2020 31518525

Beyens I, Pouwels JL, van Driel II, et al: The effect of social media on well-being differs from adolescent to adolescent. Sci Rep 10(1):10763, 2020 32612108

Burnette CB, Kwitowski MA, Mazzeo SE: "I don't need people to tell me I'm pretty on social media": a qualitative study of social media and body image in early adolescent girls. Body Image 23:114–125, 2017 28965052

Casares DR, Binkley EE: An unfiltered look at idealized images: a social media intervention for adolescent girls. J Creat Ment Health 17(3):313–331, 2022

Cavalcante A: Tumbling into queer utopias and vortexes: experiences of LGBTQ social media users on Tumblr. J Homosex 66(12):1715–1735, 2019 30235077

Centers for Disease Control and Prevention: Youth Risk Behavior Survey: Data Summary and Trends Report (2011–2021). Atlanta, GA, Centers for Disease Control and Prevention, 2021. Available at: https://www.cdc.gov/healthyyouth/data/yrbs/pdf/yrbs_data-summary-trends_report2023_508.pdf. Accessed November 29, 2023.

Chae J: Explaining females' envy toward social media influencers. Media Psychol 21(2):246–262, 2018

Cheng J, Burke M, Davis EG: Understanding perceptions of problematic Facebook use: when people experience negative life impact and a lack of control, in Proceedings of the 2019 CHI Conference on Human Factors in Computing Systems, May 2019, pp 1–13

Clark LS: Parental mediation theory for the digital age. Commun Theory 21(4):323–343, 2011

Dolan R, Conduit J, Fahy J, et al: Social media engagement behaviour: a uses and gratifications perspective. J Strateg Mark 24(3–4):261–277, 2016

Du J, Kerkhof P, van Koningsbruggen GM: Predictors of social media self-control failure: immediate gratifications, habitual checking, ubiquity, and notifications. Cyberpsychol Behav Soc Netw 22(7):477–485, 2019 31295024

Du J, Kerkhof P, van Koningsbruggen GM: The reciprocal relationships between social media self-control failure, mindfulness and wellbeing: a longitudinal study. PLoS One 16(8):e0255648, 2021 34347832

Dweck CS: Can personality be changed? The role of beliefs in personality and change. Curr Dir Psychol Sci 17(6):391–394, 2008

Ellison NB, Steinfield C, Lampe C: The benefits of Facebook "friends": social capital and college students' use of online social network sites. Journal of Computer-Mediated Communication 12(4):1143–1168, 2007

Giumetti GW, Kowalski RM: Cyberbullying via social media and well-being. Curr Opin Psychol 45:101314, 2022 35313180

Haidt J: The dangerous experiment on teen girls. The Atlantic, November 21, 2021. Available at: https://www.theatlantic.com/ideas/archive/2021/11/facebooks-dangerous-experiment-teen-girls/620767. Accessed November 29, 2023.

Hall JA, Liu D: Social media use, social displacement, and well-being. Curr Opin Psychol 46:101339, 2022 35395533

Hancock JT, Liu SX, Luo M, et al: Social media and psychological well-being, in The Psychology of Technology: Social Science Research in the Age of Big Data. Edited by Matz SC. Washington, DC, American Psychological Association, 2022, pp 195–238

Hiebert A, Kortes-Miller K: Finding home in online community: exploring TikTok as a support for gender and sexual minority youth throughout COVID-19. J LGBT Youth 20(2):1–18, 2021

Katz R, Ogilvie S, Shaw J, et al: Gen Z, Explained: The Art of Living in a Digital Age. Chicago, IL, University of Chicago Press, 2022

Kleemans M, Daalmans S, Carbaat I, et al: Picture perfect: the direct effect of manipulated Instagram photos on body image in adolescent girls. Media Psychol 21(1):93–110, 2018

Klobuchar A, Lummings C: Nudging Users to Drive Good Experiences on Social Media Act, S. 3608, 117th Congress, 2022. Available at: https://www.govinfo.gov/app/details/BILLS-117s3608is. Accessed November 29, 2023.

Krasnova H, Widjaja T, Buxmann P, et al: Why following friends can hurt you: an exploratory investigation of the effects of envy on social networking sites among college-age users. Inf Syst Res 26(3):585–605, 2015

Lanette S, Chua PK, Hayes G, et al: How much is "too much?" The role of a smartphone addiction narrative in individuals' experience of use. Proc ACM Hum Comput Interact 2(CSCW):1–22, 2018

Lee AY, Hancock J: Social media mindsets: the impact of implicit theories about social media use on psychological well-being. Paper presented at International Communication Association, May 21–26, 2020

Lee AY, Hancock J: Social media mindsets: a new approach to understanding social media use. Open Science Framework, 2023. Available at: https://osf.io/preprints/psyarxiv/f8wny. Accessed November 29, 2023.

Lee AY, Hancock J: Social media mindsets: a new approach to understanding social media use and psychological well-being. Journal of Computer-Mediated Communication 29(1):zmad048, 2024

Lee AY, Katz R, Hancock J: The role of subjective construals on reporting and reasoning about social media use. Soc Media Soc 7(3):20563051211035350, 2021

Lee AY, Mieczkowski H, Ellison NB, et al: The algorithmic crystal: conceptualizing the self through algorithmic personalization on TikTok. Proc ACM Hum Comput Interact 6(CSCW):1–22, 2022

Lee AY, Ellison NB, Hancock J: To use or be used? The role of agency in social media use and well-being. Front Comp Sci 5:1123323, 2023

Liao M, Sundar SS: Sound of silence: does muting notifications reduce phone use? Comput Human Behav 134:107338, 2022

Liu SX, Shen Q, Hancock J: Situating parenting and technology styles within social class: social class-based phone orientations (article under review)

Livingstone S, Blum-Ross A: Parenting for a Digital Future: How Hopes and Fears About Technology Shape Children's Lives. New York, Oxford University Press, 2020

Lucero L: Safe spaces in online places: social media and LGBTQ youth. Multicult Educ Rev 9(2):117–128, 2017

Lwin MO, Panchapakesan C, Teresa J, et al: Are parents doing it right? Parent and child perspectives on parental mediation in Singapore. J Fam Commun 21(4):306–321, 2021

Masur PK, Veldhuis J, Bij de Vaate N: There is no easy answer: how the interaction of content, situation, and person shapes the effects of social media use on well-being, in The Social Media Debate. Edited by Rosen D. New York, Routledge, 2022, pp 187–202

Meier A, Reinecke L: Computer-mediated communication, social media, and mental health: a conceptual and empirical meta-review. Communication Research 48(8):1182–1209, 2021

Metherell TE, Ghai S, McCormick EM, et al: Digital access constraints predict worse mental health among adolescents during COVID-19. Sci Rep 12(1):19088, 2022 36352002

Minihan S, Orben A, Songco A, et al: Social determinants of mental health during a year of the COVID-19 pandemic. Dev Psychopathol 35(4):1701–1713, 2023 35796203

O'Day EB, Heimberg RG: Social media use, social anxiety, and loneliness: a systematic review. Comput Hum Behav Rep 3:100070, 2021

Odgers CL, Jensen MR: Annual Research Review: adolescent mental health in the digital age: facts, fears, and future directions. J Child Psychol Psychiatry 61(3):336–348, 2020 31951670

Orben A: The Sisyphean cycle of technology panics. Perspect Psychol Sci 15(5):1143–1157, 2020 32603635

Orben A, Przybylski AK: The association between adolescent well-being and digital technology use. Nat Hum Behav 3(2):173–182, 2019

Panchal U, Salazar de Pablo G, Franco M, et al: The impact of COVID-19 lockdown on child and adolescent mental health: systematic review. Eur Child Adolesc Psychiatry 32(7):1151–1177, 2023 34406494

Park J, Hallman J, Liu SX, et al: Black representation in social media well-being research: a scoping review of social media experience and psychological well-being among Black users in the United States. New Media & Society 26(3):1670–1702, 2024

Pelletier MJ, Krallman A, Adams FG, et al: One size doesn't fit all: a uses and gratifications analysis of social media platforms. J Res Interact Mark 14(2):269–284, 2020

Przybylski AK, Nguyen TVT, Law W, et al: Does taking a short break from social media have a positive effect on well-being? Evidence from three preregistered field experiments. J Technol Behav Sci 6(3):507–514, 2021

Radtke T, Apel T, Schenkel K, et al: Digital detox: an effective solution in the smartphone era? A systematic literature review. Mob Media Commun 10(2):190–215, 2022

Rideout V, Peebles A, Mann S, et al: Common Sense Census: Media Use by Tweens and Teens, 2021. San Francisco, CA, Common Sense, 2022

Sabik N, Falat J, Magagnos J: When self-worth depends on social media feedback: associations with psychological well-being. Sex Roles 82:411–421, 2020

Sánchez-Valle M, de-Frutos-Torres B, Vázquez-Barrio T: Parent's influence on acquiring critical internet skills [in Spanish]. Comunicar 25(53):103–111, 2017

Schou Andreassen C, Billieux J, Griffiths MD, et al: The relationship between addictive use of social media and video games and symptoms of psychiatric disorders: a large-scale cross-sectional study. Psychol Addict Behav 30(2):252–262, 2016 26999354

Schreurs L: Adolescents' social media literacy: a theoretical and empirical analysis of its development and empowering role in social media positivity bias effects. Doctoral dissertation, Katholieke Universiteit Leuven, Belgium, 2022

Schreurs L, Vandenbosch L: Should I post my very best self? The within-person reciprocal associations between social media literacy, positivity-biased behaviors and adolescents' self-esteem. Telemat Inform 73(1):101865, 2022

Shin W, Lwin MO: Parental mediation of children's digital media use in high digital penetration countries: perspectives from Singapore and Australia. Asian J Commun 32(4):309–326, 2022

Smith KL: The impact of media on African American adolescent mental health and behavior. Doctoral dissertation, Capella University, Minneapolis, MN, 2020

Steinfield C, Ellison NB, Lampe C, et al: Online social network sites and the concept of social capital, in Frontiers in New Media Research. Edited by Lee FL, Leung L, Qui S, et al. New York, Routledge, 2013, pp 122–138

Sun Y, Zhang Y: A review of theories and models applied in studies of social media addiction and implications for future research. Addict Behav 114:106699, 2021 33268185

Tamplin NC, McLean SA, Paxton SJ: Social media literacy protects against the negative impact of exposure to appearance ideal social media images in young adult women but not men. Body Image 26:29–37, 2018

Valkenburg PM, Piotrowski JT: Plugged In: How Media Attract and Affect Youth. New Haven, CT, Yale University Press, 2017

Valkenburg PM, Meier A, Beyens I: Social media use and its impact on adolescent mental health: an umbrella review of the evidence. Curr Opin Psychol 44:58–68, 2022 34563980

Van den Bulck J, Custers K, Nelissen S: The child-effect in the new media environment: challenges and opportunities for communication research. J Child Media 10(1):30–38, 2016

Van der Stuyf RR: Scaffolding as a teaching strategy. Adolescent Learning and Development 52(3):5–18, 2002

Walther JB: Social media and online hate. Curr Opin Psychol 45:101298, 2022 35158213

Wells G, Horwitz J, Seetharaman D: Facebook knows Instagram is toxic for teen girls, company documents show. The Wall Street Journal, September 14, 2021

Yang CC, Holden SM, Ariati J: Social media and psychological well-being among youth: the multidimensional model of social media use. Clin Child Fam Psychol Rev 24(3):631–650, 2021 34169391

Yeager DS, Dweck CS: Mindsets that promote resilience: when students believe that personal characteristics can be developed. Educ Psychol 47(4):302–314, 2012

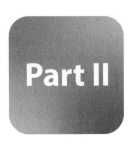

Clinical Considerations and Special Populations

8

Social Media and Adolescent Mental Health

Clinical Implications and Approaches

Zhiying Yue, Ph.D.
Michael Tsappis, M.D.
Michael Carter, Ph.D.
Fatima Bilal Motiwala, M.D.
Dalton Bourke, M.D.
Emily Izenman, B.A.
David S. Bickham, Ph.D.
Michael Rich, M.D., M.P.H.

In this chapter, we focus on the relationships among adolescents' social media use, their mental health and well-being, and relevant clinical practices by reviewing three major questions: 1) How can social media use affect well-being? 2) What is problematic interactive media use (PIMU)? and 3) How can we promote healthy social media use practices to facilitate positive health outcomes?

Family Digital Wellness Guide is available at https://digitalwellnesslab.org/family-digital-wellness-guide.

As young people enter adolescence and their social support systems en-
large and shift to include increasingly important peers, they are drawn to social media and to interactive digital technologies because these platforms
provide instant, wide-ranging access to their growing social networks and
parasocial connections. Given the prominent place that social media has
come to occupy in the lives of adolescents, it is important to understand the
potential opportunities for and risks to adolescents' mental health with regard to its use.

The term *social media* generally refers to an ever-evolving set of interactive media applications (apps) that allow for the exchange of user-generated
content by means of an internet connection (Kaplan and Haenlein 2010).
Notably, the distinctions between traditional social network sites and other
forms of interactive media are increasingly blurred. Established social media platforms have evolved, and new apps and websites have emerged that
offer varying features and functions spanning social networking, gaming,
image-sharing, and even the exchange of sexually explicit materials (Carter
et al. 2022).

Social Media Use: A Double-Edged Sword

Social media use is now an integral element of the adolescent experience because it provides an open and enriching environment for accomplishing the
key tasks of this developmental stage, such as connecting with others, exploring one's identity, seeking new life experiences, and establishing autonomy (Rich et al. 2017). Teens themselves describe social media platforms as
tools for deepening relationships, being creative, and learning more about
the world (Anderson et al. 2022). Indeed, more than 35% of American adolescents ages 13–17 report that they are "almost constantly" using at least
one of the top five online platforms: YouTube, TikTok, Instagram, Snapchat,
and Facebook (Vogels et al. 2022). Fully 83% of a nationally diverse adolescent sample ($N=1,480$) reported that they were "slightly" to "completely"
addicted to screen media (Bickham et al. 2022).

Using social media can benefit adolescents in several ways. It enables
them to stay connected with existing friends and family, make new connections, and engage in innovative activities (Anderson et al. 2022). This was
both essential and accelerated during the coronavirus disease 2019 (COVID-
19) pandemic lockdowns, when measures such as stay-at-home orders and
school closures boosted adolescents' social media use (Rideout et al. 2022).
Research shows that interactive social media use can be inversely associated
with depression and anxiety (Seabrook et al. 2016) due to the expansion of

social support, long considered crucial for psychological well-being (Meng et al. 2017). Because social media provides a low-cost way for people to maintain relationships, adolescents can feasibly broadcast messages to their entire network and use "lightweight" features (e.g., likes, reactions) to show affection that dissolves geographical distances (Carr et al. 2016). As adolescents feel greater freedom and autonomy to share personal information online versus offline, self-disclosure on social media can elicit supportive responses even from strangers while also leaving them vulnerable to "trolling" and other negative responses (Kross et al. 2021).

> I do my homework, hang out with friends, and watch videos on screen media. I'm not bored when I'm gaming.
> —*anonymous male, age 13*

Benefits associated with social media use are often accompanied by potential risks (Keles et al. 2020). Social media use has been associated with a range of mental health issues, including depression, anxiety, poor emotional regulation, diminished cognitive function, lower life satisfaction, and body dissatisfaction, as well as physical health issues including sleep disturbances/excessive daytime sleepiness, musculoskeletal problems, weight gain, vision problems, and weakened immunity (Goodyear and Armour 2019).

Social comparison, defined as evaluating one's own attributes in relation to those of others, can help explain the detrimental effect of social media use on mental health (Yue et al. 2022). Social comparison is part of normative development for adolescents; as their bodies and emotions rapidly change, they become more self-conscious and seek acceptance of their appearance and ideas. Confronted in social media with a high volume of optimized, often manipulated self-presentation by their peers, they can feel inadequate, dissatisfied, incompetent, and jealous, emotions frequently associated with poorer well-being (Nesi and Prinstein 2015). The relationship between social media–based comparisons and poorer well-being (e.g., depressive symptoms, body dissatisfaction) appears to be stronger among teenage females than teenage males (Ho et al. 2016).

Many young people take their phones to bed with them, interfering with their quantity and quality of sleep (Bickham et al. 2022). During the night, blue light from screens can suppress the release of melatonin, delaying sleep latency and reducing both the duration and quality of sleep (Cain and Gradisar 2010). Incoming alerts and notifications can disrupt drowsiness and interrupt sleep (Garrison et al. 2011). Adolescents may struggle to relax at bedtime due to emotional arousal from social media content or the fear of missing out (FOMO) on messages/posts (Scott et al. 2019). Insufficient sleep, in turn, has been associated with lower well-being and poorer health among adolescents (Zhang et al. 2017).

A global study (N=180,919) conducted across 42 countries showed that social media use was positively correlated with both the perpetration and victimization of cyberbullying (Craig et al. 2020). *Cyberbullying* is defined as intentional, aggressive acts performed by individuals or groups using digital platforms to threaten or inflict harm and discomfort on victims (Smith et al. 2008). Empirical research appears to show a significant increase in the prevalence of cyberbullying over the past 5 years, although overall prevalence rates have varied from 6.0% to 57.5%, with significant divergence in definition, measurement, and sampling (Zhu et al. 2021). In general, it is easy to find and retrieve information about a cyberbullying target on social media (Chan et al. 2019). On sites that allow greater anonymity, perpetrators can easily edit or delete their posts to deny their involvement in cyberbullying (Barlett et al. 2018). Victims of cyberbullying have more school absences, are at higher risk for depression (Gámez-Guadix et al. 2013), and are more likely to have suicidal thoughts or attempts (Arnon et al. 2022).

Previous research has suggested that active social interaction on social media is linked with positive impacts on youth's well-being, whereas passive browsing and scrolling have been associated with negative effects (Dienlin and Johannes 2020). However, more recent research has challenged the passive-active use hypothesis and highlighted the personalized nature of social media effects (Valkenburg et al. 2021). Factors such as individual characteristics, types of social interactions, aspects of the social media environment, and the use experience can all influence the strength and pattern of these effects (Beyens et al. 2020; Valkenburg et al. 2021). As a result, the impact of social media use on well-being likely varies from person to person, and it is important to consider the nuanced and personalized nature of social media effects.

Although there is rising public and policymaker concern that social media use may cause mental health problems for young people, the reality is more nuanced. The various forms of online interactive media—from traditional social networking sites (Facebook, Twitter) to social gaming (Roblox, Minecraft), image and video sharing (Snapchat, Instagram, YouTube), and blog/discussion sites on subjects of shared interest (Reddit, Quora)—represent the "village square" for many youth. These platforms are where they meet old friends and make new ones, where they compete and collaborate, where they show off and where they confess, where they hook up and where they break up. Most youth are on social media, and most are all right. Like it or not, in the "next normal," interactive media might be essential to success in education, employment, communication, entertainment, and connection with others.

Adolescence is a time of great change physically, cognitively, and emotionally. There is excitement and anxiety, exhilaration and sadness, hope and despair. As a primary place where youth meet, social media does not *create* anxiety or depression, but it can enable and amplify the powerful emotions of adolescence. Some young people take refuge in social media, living out their emotions, hopes, and dreams in what they perceive to be a protected environment, but they then suffer because the environment is not as emotionally safe as they had hoped and because they spend time on social media at the expense of a more diversified and physically, mentally, and socially healthy lifestyle.

Problematic Interactive Media Use

A minority of adolescents experience unique challenges with social media use which can result in academic failure, social withdrawal, behavioral problems, family conflict, and physical and mental health problems (Paakkari et al. 2021). Early concern about interactive online behaviors becoming dysfunctional led to a proposed diagnosis of *internet addiction* in the 1990s (Young 1998). Focusing on interactive gaming as problematic behavior, the American Psychiatric Association proposed *internet gaming disorder* as a potential diagnosis that required further study in DSM-5 (American Psychiatric Association 2013). In 2019, the World Health Organization included *gaming disorder* as a diagnosis in their *International Classification of Diseases,* 11th Revision (ICD-11; World Health Organization 2019). Although these descriptions represent needed progress toward characterizing dysfunctional gaming, criteria vary among them and do not account for other manifestations of PIMU.

Between November 2017 and December 2022, the Clinic for Interactive Media and Internet Disorders (CIMAID) at Boston Children's Hospital evaluated and cared for 338 youth whose use of online interactive sites resulted in functional physical, mental, or social impairment. Clinical experience from CIMAID has demonstrated that children and adolescents present with one or more of four dysregulated behaviors on computers, consoles, tablets, and/or smartphones: social media use; gaming (online or offline); pornography use; and information bingeing on news, discussion, and/or short-form video aggregators (Pluhar et al. 2019).

> I don't know how much time I am gaming— I lose track of
> it. When they tell me to stop, it pisses me off, because I'm
> not done, and I don't think I've been on as long as they do.
> I can't stand it when they make me do homework or go to
> bed instead.
>
> *—anonymous male, age 12*

It is crucial to distinguish between the "new normal" experienced by most young people in the digital ecosystem and the dysregulation of interactive media use that poses a risk to physical, mental, and social health. We propose that *social media* has become an increasingly unclear genre because most online activities now include a social component: networking, dating, information-seeking, gaming, blogging, and so on. *Interactive media* could be a more unifying description that focuses on *interactivity* and its variable rewards as the key to user engagement. Over the past several decades, researchers have revealed troubling use of interactive media across a wide variety of devices, platforms, and apps, yielding more than 100 names for this condition depending on what the researcher was studying (of which 14 specifically name social media). Interactivity is the common thread in all of these cases and, in our clinical experience, the more relevant focus of inquiry than a specific technology, game, or app.

Although problematic social media use was the most prevalent chief complaint among young females and problematic gaming was the most prevalent chief complaint among young males, most CIMAID patients revealed that they moved fluidly among multiple devices, platforms, and types of interactive media use, online and offline. When they lost access to their smartphones, they continued their social media use on computers. When they lost their internet connection, they gamed offline. When they were restricted from gaming, they video-streamed others' gaming or talked about gaming on social media. Their intense engagement was not with specific devices or apps but with the interactivity (in most cases with online or offline friends and peers). Naming the issue *internet addiction* or *gaming disorder* points to the technology, rather than the use of it, as the source of the problem. Because these behaviors are not limited to specific activities, devices, or platforms, we have found a comprehensive and accurate nomenclature for this condition to be *problematic interactive media use*, which focuses on the dysregulated use behaviors of the person rather than on the specific technology, platform, or app being used.

Patients' self-efficacy is discounted when they believe or are told that they are not in control of their behavior, which can lead to denial and make acceptance/recovery more difficult (Rich et al. 2017). In our culture, labeling something as an addiction can be stigmatizing, blaming the "addict" as weak or immoral. Parents of a child with PIMU may not see them as being "addicted" until the child has become seriously impaired. This delay in identification may lead to avoidance or further delay in seeking necessary care (Fraser et al. 2017). While internet or video game addiction terminology used in earlier research drew needed attention to problematic behaviors with interactive media, use of *addiction* has been criticized as both biomedically inaccurate and culturally stigmatizing (Panova and Carbonell 2018; Rich et al. 2017). Substance use disorder or addiction is characterized by the use of a pleasurable but unnecessary substance (e.g., alcohol, opioids) that causes measurable, reproducible biological changes during use and withdrawal from use, and the treatment for this is abstinence. In contrast, PIMU, although not classified as a behavioral disorder, shares similarities with binge eating disorder (BED) in terms of the underlying mechanisms. Both PIMU and BED involve the overuse of a necessary resource (i.e., interactive media vs. food) driven by unmet psychological needs that continues despite negative consequences and results in physical, mental, or social dysfunction. Treatment strategies for both PIMU and BED focus on self-regulation and more effective use of that necessary resource rather than abstinence.

> I don't think social media is bad for my health—actually, I have made friends and stayed connected through COVID. It's not social media that's the problem, it's how some people use it that screws them up.
> —*anonymous male, age 18*

Consistent with the paper by Piotrowski and Valkenburg (2015), we have found that young people have different susceptibilities to the effects of media use. For example, adolescents with ADHD are more likely to struggle with dysfunctional media use than are neurotypical youth (Settanni et al. 2018). A study with 100 youth, 50 neurotypical and 50 with ADHD, found that those with ADHD were 9.3 times more likely to struggle with PIMU (Enagandula et al. 2018). The dopamine deficit theory proposes that, compared with neurotypical children, young people with ADHD are driven by gratification with smaller and more immediate—rather than delayed—

rewards (Tripp and Wickens 2008). For youth whose attentional difficulties make them feel inadequate in the classroom and in social situations, the relentless stimulation and variable rewards of interactive media, whether they be points in gaming (e.g., in-game currency and experience points) or the receipt of views and likes, can be soothing, satisfying, and empowering.

Autism spectrum disorder (ASD) was also identified in a clinical sample as an underlying diagnosis evident in more than 40% of young people with dysregulated interactive media use (Kawabe et al. 2019). Online communication platforms, such as massively multiplayer online games and the asynchronous venue of social media, offer less threatening, easier-to-understand social environments for adolescents with ASD who desire human connection but often have deficits in social skills (Pluhar et al. 2019). Rather than devices, platforms, or apps *causing* mental health problems, young people with underlying mental health issues appear to be immersing themselves in interactive media to distract themselves from their primary discomfort and to soothe themselves with their mastery of the digital environment.

Anxiety and depression are prevalent among CIMAID patients (Bickham 2021). Youth with anxiety, particularly social anxiety, are drawn to social media in their desire to make connections in a space they perceive to be "safe." Depressed youth may gravitate to social media because the platforms allow them to escape from the "real world," relieve stress, express aggression, and demonstrate competence in ways they fear to attempt offline (Cudo et al. 2022; Keles et al. 2020; Radovic et al. 2017). Unfortunately, using social media can often exacerbate anxiety and depression due to the effects of social comparison, "trolling," cyberbullying, solicitation of sexts, and even sexual predation (Kross et al. 2021; O'Keeffe et al. 2011).

The recognition of underlying psychological issues in patients and our observation that PIMU may decrease, disappear, or be more easily managed with behavioral modification when these problems are effectively treated lead us to view it as a syndrome in which the signs and symptoms of a person's underlying condition manifest themselves in the interactive media environment. The repetitive use of interactive media across different types of devices and platforms may be initiated to distract, self-soothe, and feel better. However, it can become problematic when it displaces sleep, nutrition, physical activities, academic work, and school attendance; disrupts relationships with family and friends; and impairs the person's physical, mental, cognitive, or social functions. PIMU can occur in someone who experiences anxiety or other psychological struggles but who does not necessarily meet the diagnostic criteria for any specific disorder. In this sense, it can be seen as a maladaptive coping strategy that can impair individuals as much or more than the underlying situation being coped with.

It is essential to understand that mental health issues are not binary, or simple "yes/no" categories; instead, conditions such as anxiety, depression, ADHD, and ASD exist on a continuum of severity. Virtually everyone encounters various forms of emotional stress and psychological challenges at different points in their lives, stemming from a wide range of sources, including personal, social, and environmental factors. Thus, it is not solely the presence or absence of a specific diagnosis that matters but, rather, the individual's psychological state and their ability to cope with the challenges they face.

Given this perspective, assessing and treating PIMU requires a comprehensive approach that considers the underlying conditions that may be contributing to the problematic use, such as an adolescent's psychological needs and conditions, executive functioning, and family environment (Brand et al. 2016). Notably, PIMU can be habituated and persist even when the underlying conditions are better managed. Therefore, adolescents often need behavioral modification to manage dysfunctional PIMU behaviors because their executive functions of self-regulation and impulse control are not yet fully developed. It is vital both to address the underlying conditions and to implement behavioral modification strategies that include active participation of parents, educators, and the adolescents themselves. Neglecting the complex nature of PIMU, either by focusing solely on the underlying condition or on behavioral modification, may not result in comprehensive and enduring improvement. In the following section, we discuss strategies for regulating adolescents' media use to support their overall well-being.

Promoting Healthy Social Media Use Practices

Understanding the media use expectations within individual families is crucial for establishing healthy media practices for young people. It is important to recognize that what is considered "normal" may vary based on familial and cultural values. In general, parental engagement plays a critical role in fostering responsible media use (Chen and Shi 2018). Parents are encouraged to provide sound guidance and to model intentional media use from the child's infancy, to establish and uphold household rules centered on content and communication, and to introduce their children to media tools when necessary, ensuring that they can manage those devices and apps responsibly (Moreno et al. 2022).

Early adolescence (ages 10–13 years) is a pivotal time for active parenting with respect to a child's interactive media use. Developmentally, children are seeking greater autonomy from their parents and greater connection with their peers. This is the time when most will ask for and receive smartphones and social media accounts. Active mentoring and using new devices and apps together when introducing them provides a foundation for their use. Establishing clear expectations about which interactive platforms the youth will use and when and how they will use them protects against future confusion and conflict. There is no automatic assumption of a right to privacy for the adolescent who is still a decade removed from full executive function. This is about biology, not discrimination. Adolescents do not have a fully developed prefrontal cortex until their mid- to late twenties, which can impact their understanding of privacy and its future implications. Parents may support their children in navigating the online world by setting up social media and gaming accounts together and by checking in every now and then to see how their children are faring. By maintaining open communication, parents can help youth feel supported and provide guidance when needed (Reid Chassiakos et al. 2016).

By sharing their child's media experiences, learning from their natural facility with the technology, and providing a counterbalance of executive function, parents can support their child's mental health and effective media use rather than policing the latter. We advise parents to avoid overreacting to unhealthy online experiences but, rather, to remain calm and to capitalize on "teachable moments." As adolescents mature and develop their digital citizenship, parents can gradually decrease their oversight of the child's activities and increase the child's access to devices, apps, and communications that might be more private. Meta-analytical results show that prohibiting or limiting the use of media can decrease children's overuse, but co-viewing (using media with the child) and active mediation (discussing and explaining media with the child) are also associated with decreased rates of adverse media use outcomes (Chen and Shi 2018).

I have a lot of friends, some nearby, some far away. I stay in touch with them on Snapchat and Instagram, and I text with them. But my parents are unfair to restrict my media use. My younger sister has more media and less limitations. I don't have a problem overusing media. My phone has been taken away a couple times, and I've handled it.

—anonymous female, age 15

Although there is parental and public concern about potential negative effects of interactive media use, effective care for adolescents requires the clinician to maintain a balanced perspective in order to help the youth navigate negative experiences online and offline and guide them toward positive media use and outcomes. Adolescents strive for autonomy and freedom; they are more resistant to guidance and care if their normative desire for connection and communication on social media is consistently blamed as harmful. A neutral, accepting stance toward interactive media serves to build alliances, allows conversations about young people's social media successes and challenges, and offers opportunities to process these experiences with their clinicians.

Clinical evaluation of media effects should be included in standard-of-care comprehensive health assessments of children and adolescents, including a longitudinal developmental history; mental health symptoms and treatment history; medical, family, and social history; and safety assessment and intervention plans as indicated. Youth often lack insight regarding their media use, so building an alliance with them and making efforts to enhance their motivation, starting from the first greeting and assessment, can help them gain needed perspective. Clinicians should ask about the adolescent's media use history and use patterns through the course of development, focusing not only on amount of use but also on motivations for use, positive and negative use experiences, and the interplay between use and the family environment. In doing so, the clinician monitors for themes and patterns that provide clues to the functions of the youth's media use behaviors, along with any biopsychosocial factors that impart risk for or protection against PIMU (Rich et al. 2017). Note that an accurate and comprehensive assessment of PIMU requires thorough investigation into the youth's interactive media use behaviors and their social, mental, and physical functioning, as well as their medical and psychological history. Only by collectively examining the child's psychiatric conditions, overall mental and physical health, and social relationships, as well as their media use, can clinicians get a better understanding of the presence and development of PIMU.

Several established psychotherapeutic approaches have been shown to be effective in regulating adolescents' media use. Cognitive-behavioral therapy (CBT) involves self-monitoring, identifying potential denial about maladaptive patterns of media use, and cognitive restructuring of any thought distortions (e.g., dichotomous thinking) that promote impulsive media use behaviors (Young 2013). CBT can identify and reconstruct the cognitive and behavioral sphere that supported the development of PIMU, allowing individuals to develop healthier, more adaptive media use habits and skills (Lopez-Fernandez et al. 2022). Although empirical studies on CBT as a tool to address PIMU are still scarce, it has been shown that CBT can reduce the obsessive-compulsive symptoms found in PIMU, as well as any associated psychological and psychopathological symptoms (Stevens et al. 2019; Wölfling et al. 2014).

Family counseling can also significantly reduce the severity of PIMU among adolescents (Young and de Abreu 2017). Family interventions involve the collaborative development of a media plan with explicit, highly specific expectations of the parent(s) and adolescent. Such plans represent goals, not orders, to be followed by both parents and children. Nonadherence motivates collaborative discussion between the clinician and the family to refine their formulation of the problem and inform future courses of treatment. The goals of an effective media plan include developing agreement between parents and adolescents to regulate intentional media use; encouraging adolescents' self-control and clearly communicating the consequences for not meeting the expectations; and avoiding abrupt and unexpected parental directives, such as immediate cessation of media use, that can escalate family conflicts. When deviations from media plans occur, families and children are encouraged to bring their concerns to their next clinical appointment instead of arguing in the moment, which helps maintain safety and mutual trust in a potentially volatile situation.

Conclusion

Given the ubiquity of interactive media, there are ongoing public and private debates about adolescents' media use and how it relates to their well-being. Our digital ecosystem provides another fertile environment for adolescent development, with nearly unlimited opportunities for learning; broadening exposure to people, cultures, and experiences; establishing independence; exploring identity; seeking connections; and building community. PIMU can negatively affect well-being by disrupting sleep, nutrition, academic performance, and physical activities; interfering with family and friend relationships; exposing youth to cyberbullying and risky sexual behavior; and amplifying anxiety and depression. Importantly, it has now been recognized as a public health issue. To effectively prevent, recognize, and treat the signs and symptoms and underlying factors associated with PIMU, child and adolescent clinicians must work together with parents and educators to standardize nomenclature, assessment, and treatment strategies for PIMU and underlying conditions. Despite the risks, interactive media are now both inevitable and an essential part of adolescent development. Today's youth on social media are tomorrow's adults, using their twenty-first-century skills to imagine, innovate, and produce the future.

References

Anderson M, Vogels EA, Perrin A, et al: Connection, creativity and drama: teen life on social media in 2022. Pew Research Center, November 16, 2022. Available at: https://www.pewresearch.org/internet/2022/11/16/connection-creativity-and-drama-teen-life-on-social-media-in-2022. Accessed November 30, 2023.

American Psychiatric Association: Diagnostic and Statistical Manual of Mental Disorders, 5th Edition. Arlington, VA, American Psychiatric Association, 2013

Arnon S, Brunstein Klomek A, Visoki E, et al: Association of cyberbullying experiences and perpetration with suicidality in early adolescence. JAMA Netw Open 5(6):e2218746, 2022 35759263

Barlett CP, DeWitt CC, Maronna B, et al: Social media use as a tool to facilitate or reduce cyberbullying perpetration: a review focusing on anonymous and nonanonymous social media platforms. Violence Gend 5(3):147–152, 2018

Beyens I, Pouwels JL, van Driel II, et al: The effect of social media on well-being differs from adolescent to adolescent. Sci Rep 10(1):10763, 2020 32612108

Bickham DS: Current research and viewpoints on internet addiction in adolescents. Curr Pediatr Rep 9(1):1–10, 2021 33457108

Bickham D, Hunt E, Bediou B, et al: Adolescent Media Use: Attitudes, Effects, and Online Experiences. Boston, MA, Boston Children's Hospital Digital Wellness Lab, August 2022. Available at: https://digitalwellnesslab.org/wp-content/uploads/Pulse-Survey_Adolescent-Attitudes-Effects-and-Experiences.pdf. Accessed November 30, 2023.

Brand M, Young KS, Laier C, et al: Integrating psychological and neurobiological considerations regarding the development and maintenance of specific internet-use disorders: an Interaction of Person-Affect-Cognition-Execution (I-PACE) model. Neurosci Biobehav Rev 71(December):252–266, 2016 27590829

Cain N, Gradisar M: Electronic media use and sleep in school-aged children and adolescents: a review. Sleep Med 11(8):735–742, 2010 20673649

Carr CT, Wohn DY, Hayes RA: As social support: relational closeness, automaticity, and interpreting social support from paralinguistic digital affordances in social media. Comput Human Behav 62(September):385–393, 2016

Carter MC, Cingel DP, Ruiz JB, et al: Social media use in the context of the personal social media ecosystem framework. J Commun 73(1):25–37, 2022

Chan TKH, Cheung CMK, Wong RYM: Cyberbullying on social networking sites: the crime opportunity and affordance perspectives. J Manage Inf Syst 36(2):574–609, 2019

Chen L, Shi J: Reducing harm from media: a meta-analysis of parental mediation. Journalism & Mass Communication Quarterly 96(1):173–193, 2018

Craig W, Boniel-Nissim M, King N, et al: Social media use and cyber-bullying: a cross-national analysis of young people in 42 countries. J Adolesc Health 66(6S):S100–S108, 2020 32446603

Cudo A, Dobosz M, Griffiths MD, et al: The relationship between early maladaptive schemas, depression, anxiety, and problematic video gaming among female and male gamers. Int J Ment Health Addict (July):1–28, 2022 35789815

Dienlin T, Johannes N: The impact of digital technology use on adolescent well-being? Dialogues Clin Neurosci 22(2):135–142, 2020 32699513

Enagandula R, Singh S, Adgaonkar GW, et al: Study of internet addiction in children with attention-deficit hyperactivity disorder and normal control. Ind Psychiatry J 27(1):110–114, 2018 30416301

Fraser S, Pienaar K, Dilkes-Frayne E, et al: Addiction stigma and the biopolitics of liberal modernity: a qualitative analysis. Int J Drug Policy 44(June):192–201, 2017 28366599

Gámez-Guadix M, Orue I, Smith PK, et al: Longitudinal and reciprocal relations of cyberbullying with depression, substance use, and problematic internet use among adolescents. J Adolesc Health 53(4):446–452, 2013 23721758

Garrison MM, Liekweg K, Christakis DA: Media use and child sleep: the impact of content, timing, and environment. Pediatrics 128(1):29–35, 2011 21708803

Goodyear VA, Armour KM: Young People, Social Media, and Health. New York, Routledge, 2019

Ho SS, Lee EWJ, Liao Y: Social network sites, friends, and celebrities: the roles of social comparison and celebrity involvement in adolescents' body image dissatisfaction. Soc Media Soc 2(3):205630511666421, 2016

Kaplan AM, Haenlein M: Users of the world, unite! The challenges and opportunities of social media. Bus Horiz 53(1):59–68, 2010

Kawabe K, Horiuchi F, Miyama T, et al: Internet addiction and attention-deficit/hyperactivity disorder symptoms in adolescents with autism spectrum disorder. Res Dev Disabil 89(June):22–28, 2019 30877993

Keles B, McCrae N, Grealish A: A systematic review: the influence of social media on depression, anxiety and psychological distress in adolescents. Int J Adolesc Youth 25(1):79–93, 2020

Kross E, Verduyn P, Sheppes G, et al: Social media and well-being: pitfalls, progress, and next steps. Trends Cogn Sci 25(1):55–66, 2021 33187873

Lopez-Fernandez O, Romo L, Kern L, et al: Perceptions underlying addictive technology use patterns: insights for cognitive-behavioural therapy. Int J Environ Res Public Health 19(1):544, 2022 35010804

Meng J, Martinez L, Holmstrom A, et al: Research on social networking sites and social support from 2004 to 2015: a narrative review and directions for future research. Cyberpsychol Behav Soc Netw 20(1):44–51, 2017 28002686

Moreno MA, Binger K, Zhao Q, et al: Digital technology and media use by adolescents: latent class analysis. JMIR Pediatr Parent 5(2):e35540, 2022 35507401

Nesi J, Prinstein MJ: Using social media for social comparison and feedback-seeking: gender and popularity moderate associations with depressive symptoms. J Abnorm Child Psychol 43(8):1427–1438, 2015 25899879

O'Keeffe GS, Clarke-Pearson K, Council on Communications and Media: The impact of social media on children, adolescents, and families. Pediatrics 127(4):800–804, 2011 21444588

Paakkari L, Tynjälä J, Lahti H, et al: Problematic social media use and health among adolescents. Int J Environ Res Public Health 18(4):1885, 2021 33672074

Panova T, Carbonell X: Is smartphone addiction really an addiction? J Behav Addict 7(2):252–259, 2018 29895183

Piotrowski JT, Valkenburg PM: Finding orchids in a field of dandelions. Am Behav Sci 59(14):1776–1789, 2015

Pluhar E, Kavanaugh JR, Levinson JA, et al: Problematic interactive media use in teens: comorbidities, assessment, and treatment. Psychol Res Behav Manag 12(June):447–455, 2019 31308769

Radovic A, Gmelin T, Stein BD, et al: Depressed adolescents' positive and negative use of social media. J Adolesc 55(55):5–15, 2017 27997851

Reid Chassiakos YL, Radesky J, Christakis D, et al: Children and adolescents and digital media. Pediatrics 138(5):e20162593, 2016 27940795

Rich M, Tsappis M, Kavanaugh JR: Problematic interactive media use among children and adolescents: addiction, compulsion, or syndrome? in Internet Addiction in Children and Adolescents: Risk Factors, Assessment, and Treatment. Edited by Young KS, de Abreu CN. New York, Springer, 2017, pp 3–28

Rideout V, Peebles A, Mann S, et al: The Common Sense Census: Media Use by Tweens and Teens. Common Sense Media, 2022. Available at: https://www.commonsensemedia.org/sites/default/files/research/report/8-18-census-integrated-report-final-web_0.pdf. Accessed November 30, 2023.

Scott H, Biello SM, Woods HC: Identifying drivers for bedtime social media use despite sleep costs: the adolescent perspective. Sleep Health 5(6):539–545, 2019 31523005

Seabrook EM, Kern ML, Rickard NS: Social networking sites, depression, and anxiety: a systematic review. JMIR Ment Health 3(4):e50, 2016 27881357

Settanni M, Marengo D, Fabris MA, et al: The interplay between ADHD symptoms and time perspective in addictive social media use: a study on adolescent Facebook users. Child Youth Serv Rev 89(June):165–170, 2018

Smith PK, Mahdavi J, Carvalho M, et al: Cyberbullying: its nature and impact in secondary school pupils. J Child Psychol Psychiatry 49(4):376–385, 2008 18363945

Stevens MWR, King DL, Dorstyn D, et al: Cognitive-behavioral therapy for internet gaming disorder: a systematic review and meta-analysis. Clin Psychol Psychother 26(2):191–203, 2019 30341981

Tripp G, Wickens JR: Research review: dopamine transfer deficit: a neurobiological theory of altered reinforcement mechanisms in ADHD. J Child Psychol Psychiatry 49(7):691–704, 2008 18081766

Valkenburg PM, van Driel II, Beyens I: The associations of active and passive social media use with well-being: a critical scoping review. New Media Soc 24(2):146144482110654, 2021

Vogels EA, Gelles-Watnick R, Massarat N: Teens, social media and technology 2022. Pew Research Center, August 10, 2022. Available at: https://www.pewresearch.org/internet/2022/08/10/teens-social-media-and-technology-2022. Accessed November 30, 2023.

Wölfling K, Beutel ME, Dreier M, et al: Treatment outcomes in patients with internet addiction: a clinical pilot study on the effects of a cognitive-behavioral therapy program. BioMed Res Int 2014:425924, 2014 25097858

World Health Organization: International Statistical Classification of Diseases and Related Health Problems, 11th Revision. Geneva, World Health Organization, 2019

Young K: Internet addiction: the emergence of a new clinical disorder. Cyberpsychol Behav 1(3):237–244, 1998

Young KS: Treatment outcomes using CBT-IA with internet-addicted patients. J Behav Addict 2(4):209–215, 2013 25215202

Young KS, de Abreu CN (eds): Internet Addiction in Children and Adolescents: Risk Factors, Assessment, and Treatment. New York, Springer, 2017

Yue Z, Zhang R, Xiao J: Passive social media use and psychological well-being during the COVID-19 pandemic: the role of social comparison and emotion regulation. Comput Human Behav 127(February):107050, 2022 34646057

Zhang J, Paksarian D, Lamers F, et al: Sleep patterns and mental health correlates in US adolescents. J Pediatr 182(March):137–143, 2017 27939122

Zhu C, Huang S, Evans R, et al: Cyberbullying among adolescents and children: a comprehensive review of the global situation, risk factors, and preventive measures. Front Public Health 9(March):634909, 2021 33791270

9

Media Multitasking, Social Media, and the Developing Brain

Impacts on Attention, Memory, and Brain Processing

Wisnu Wiradhany, Ph.D.
Susanne Baumgartner, Ph.D.

Our aim in this chapter is to provide an overview of the current findings from studies that investigated the effects of social media and media multitasking on cognitive processing. We start by (re)introducing the mechanisms by which people attend, regulate, and process incoming information in the brain. We apply these mechanisms to social media–related information processing using short illustrations. We then provide an overview of the existing studies on the effects of social media and media multitasking during task performance and the potential long-term effects of media multitasking on cognition and academic performance. We conclude by discussing the societal and clinical implications of social media for cognitive processing and academic performance.

"Check this out!" A notification pops up on our phone. We suddenly become more alert, and our attention gets automatically directed to our device.

At the same time, we might abandon the task at hand to attend to the message. Social media, for better or worse, has permeated our everyday lives to such an extent that researchers have introduced the term *permanently online/permanently connected* (PO/PC) to describe our relationship with it (Vorderer et al. 2018). Particularly, 46% of U.S. teens reported that they used the internet "almost constantly" (Vogels et al. 2022). Given this almost constant interaction between people and media, media distractions might occur frequently during the day.

Social media is particularly attractive to youth (Vogels et al. 2022). One reason for this is that young people strive for social exploration as part of their developmental trajectory (Rothbart and Rueda 2005). However, the malleability of their brains also means that they might be particularly vulnerable to the negative effects of social media. This is especially true because interactions with social media are seamlessly interleaved in our everyday activities, a phenomenon we refer to as *media multitasking* (Wiradhany et al. 2021). Researchers have suggested that continuous switches from our tasks at hand to our social media may alter how we process information for the worse (Lin 2009; Uncapher et al. 2017). Accordingly, the number of studies investigating the impact of social media on attention, memory, and brain processing has substantially increased since the early 2000s (see, e.g., Appel et al. 2020 for a meta-analysis). Yet empirical findings have been mixed, and the social and clinical implications of these studies are still being debated.

How Do Social Media and Media Multitasking Affect Information Processing?

Social media is designed to attract and engage users' attention via continuous streams of information from fellow users, content creators, and business institutions (Bayer et al. 2020). When users' attention is attracted involuntarily, social media *distractions* occur, which may lead to derailment of an ongoing train of thought and decreased productivity. Fortunately, the mechanisms under which attention is directed and redirected from one event or task to another are relatively well understood. Understanding these mechanisms helps researchers and practitioners alike identify boundary conditions under which social media distractions occur (e.g., Brasel and Gips 2017) and provides insights to help develop better interventions that prevent or reduce the harmful effects of these distractions (e.g., Martini et al. 2020).

Imagine a teenager doing their homework when a smartphone notification comes in, indicated by a notification sound. As a direct consequence of the notification, the teenager might check their phone. To the teenager, this checking behavior might seem almost automatic and effortless. However, at the cognitive level, this incoming message actually triggers three relatively independent attention systems that correspond to an increase in the teenager's level of arousal, a diversion of their gaze from their computer screen to their smartphone, and, depending on how important the message was, a decision to resist the temptation to immediately check the message. These three events correspond to *alerting*, *orienting*, and *executive attention*, respectively (Petersen and Posner 2012). First proposed in the 1990s (Posner and Petersen 1990), these attention mechanisms have been shown to be relatively independent of one another in behavioral (Fan et al. 2002) and neuroimaging studies (Aston-Jones and Cohen 2005; Botvinick and Braver 2015; Corbetta et al. 2008; Fan et al. 2005), and they develop at different ages (Mahoney et al. 2010; Mullane et al. 2016).

Attention Alerting

A sudden change in our immediate environment, such as an incoming notification, increases our level of vigilance and arousal. If we are relatively drowsy, the notification might make us more alert, which might actually help us engage with the task at hand. If we are already alert, however, the incoming notification might actually distract us from our primary task via the *attention-orienting* mechanism. These relationships correspond to the classic Yerkes-Dodson inverted-U curve (e.g., Teigen 1994): As people become stimulated from a drowsy to a moderately aroused state, their performance increases, but when stimulated from a moderately aroused to an overenergized state, their performance decreases. Infants demonstrate this so-called attention-alerting capacity between the ages of 3 months and 9 months, and it becomes well-developed during middle childhood (ages 6–9 years) (Mezzacappa 2004; Mullane et al. 2016).

The signal for attention alerting originates in our brain stem, specifically in the locus coeruleus, which produces the neurotransmitter norepinephrine (Aston-Jones and Cohen 2005). Norepinephrine may be discharged in two modes. Salient, discrete sensory stimuli—for example, if our notification was just a reminder for us to finish our homework—might elicit the short-lasting *phasic discharge* that aids a goal-directed behavior, such as finishing our homework. In contrast, salient but sustained sensory stimuli (e.g., a fire alarm) elicit a long-lasting *tonic discharge* that increases our baseline level of alertness, making us more sensitive to incoming stimuli but less able to discriminate relevant from irrelevant information. If our tonic level of alertness is already high, for example, because we have been waiting for important news from friends, the incoming notification on our phone would be more taxing to our homework performance because a high level of alertness is associated with a high level of distractibility.

Attention Orienting

The presence of a salient stimulus in our environment, such as a sound from an incoming notification and the increasing brightness of our smartphone screen in an otherwise quiet, dim room, attracts our sensory systems to a particular location or modality. This orienting behavior can already be seen in its rudimentary form in infants ages 6–9 months, and this capacity becomes well-developed during middle childhood (ages 6–9 years) (Mezzacappa 2004; Mullane et al. 2016).

Our *orienting* response is regulated by two information processing pathways. The incoming sound from a smartphone notification in our example would activate the ventral attention pathway, which regulates the exogenous form, or bottom-up attention, that involves, among others, the temporoparietal junction (Corbetta et al. 2008). This type of attention orienting is generated by external stimuli in our environment. In contrast, if we consciously check for incoming messages regularly, for instance, because we are expecting important news, the orienting behavior activates the dorsal attention pathway, which regulates the endogenous form, or top-down attention, and involves, among others, the frontal eye fields. The neurotransmitter acetylcholine modulates the orienting mechanism (Yu and Dayan 2005). In contrast to exogenous attention, this type of attention orienting is generated internally by our brain.

In everyday situations, whether *exogenous stimuli* will attract our attention *away* from our current task would depend on whether our *endogenous attention* is engaged, which we discuss further in the next section.

Executive Attention

An incoming message provides an opportunity for alternative behavior to the homework task we have at hand. Here, we are presented with a dilemma: should we stop to check the incoming message or finish the sentence we are currently writing? If we choose the latter, we trigger the inhibition of the attention mechanism, otherwise known as *executive attention* (Petersen and Posner 2012). Infants by the age of 12 months have shown rudimentary executive functioning, and this capacity is more formally developed somewhat later during childhood (ages 8–10 years) (Mezzacappa 2004; Mullane et al. 2016). Our executive function mechanism is regulated by the conflict detection and resolution part of the brain, which includes the anterior cingulate cortex (Botvinick and Braver 2015). The neurotransmitter dopamine maintains our behavior-goal contingency, therefore potentially helping us sustain our goal-directed behavior.

In sum, when social media distraction occurs, we engage three relatively independent cognitive systems. Laboratory studies have revealed important insights about these systems and have provided evidence that they work independently (Fan et al. 2002, 2005). In everyday situations, however, it is difficult to test these systems independently because an observed behavior might be the result of an interaction between them. Using our example of homework and notifications, in some cases the notification might engage all of the systems (e.g., the student decided to inhibit the notification response and stayed on task), none of the systems (e.g., the student was not aware of the notification), or some of the systems but not the others (e.g., the student responded to the notification, diverting their attention away from the homework). A better understanding of how our attention systems cooperate with one another in such situations can help researchers and practitioners recognize the circumstances under which interactions with social media help or hinder optimal cognitive processing in young people.

Effects on Cognition

The presence of the attention regulation systems in our brain indicates that we are relatively well-equipped to deal with rapid changes in our environment, adapting our behavior and changing our focus as needed. Yet one particular concern of researchers and practitioners alike is: What if social media distraction strains our information processing systems *too much?* To what extent do social media and, relatedly, media multitasking lead youth to process information more shallowly (Lin 2009; Uncapher et al. 2017)?

Observational studies have shown that media multitasking occurs at a high rate. For example, switches between a television and a computer screen occurred two times per minute (Segijn et al. 2017) to almost four times per minute (Brasel and Gips 2011, 2017), although almost half of these switches occurred for less than 1.5 seconds (Brasel and Gips 2011). In line with how our attention systems work, many of these switches were preceded by low-level visual cues such as motion and changes in luminance that triggered our reorienting function (i.e., bottom-up cues), whereas high-level visual cues such as faces or animals discouraged switching from the main task (Brasel and Gips 2017). Another observational study showed that, during a 3-hour study session, students were distracted for almost 30 minutes, mostly by social media (Calderwood et al. 2014).

These rapid rates of media multitasking somewhat negatively affect cognition and performance. Several experiments in which participants had to attend to media-related distractions while performing a primary task (e.g., retaining the contents of a lecture or a news article) showed that participants in the distracted condition performed worse. Brooks (2015), for instance, showed that the number of interactions with social media tabs in a simulated browser was negatively correlated with the amount of recalled materials from a video. In contrast, another study in which participants had to attend to advertisements presented on television, a tablet, or both showed that, in spite of their rapid rate of switching between the television and the tablet, participants could still recall the ads well (Segijn et al. 2017). Additionally, in line with the Yerkes-Dodson law (Teigen 1994), in a study in which multitasking was observed in a simulated browser, participants who multitasked a moderate amount finished a greater number of tasks compared with those who multitasked very frequently or infrequently. These varying results indicate that the relationship between media multitasking and performance might not be linear.

The negative impact of social media on performance might depend on whether it was perceived as an additional goal. For instance, incoming notifications might be distracting if the active goal is to finish one's homework but not distracting if the goal is to check and engage with social media. In a series of experiments, Szumowska and Kruglanski (2022) showed a linear relationship between active goals and multitasking. Participants switched between tasks more frequently when they had more active goals. However, prompting participants to reflect on their primary goals also reduced unnecessary multitasking. This goal-activation observation might explain why an interaction with additional (media-related) tasks sometimes may lead to worse performance (Brooks 2015) and sometimes not (Segijn et al. 2017). For instance, if our focus of attention is endogenously engaged with a task (e.g., homework), it is less likely that a notification will exogenously attract our attention.

Because youth spend a significant proportion of their time studying, most studies focused on investigating either social media engagement and media multitasking *during* learning or the correlations between media multitasking behavior and academic performance. The former showed that, in general, when multitasking occurred during learning, academic performance suffered. Downs et al. (2015), for instance, compared recall performance from a video lecture during which media multitasking could occur in a restricted or unrestricted manner. They found that unrestricted media multitasking led to worse video content recall, but restricted media multitasking (i.e., allowing participants to use their laptop or tablet to take notes) actually supported video content recall. With regard to social media use and media multitasking habits, studies have shown that increased social media use and media multitasking were associated with worse academic performance. These findings have been synthesized in meta-analyses (see Appel et al. 2020), but although these meta-analyses showed a statistically significant association between increased social media use and poor academic performance, the pooled effect size was low. Marker et al. (2018) noted that the association between social media use during academic activities and academic performance was moderated by the purpose for which social media was used. If social media were used for academic purposes during academic activities, for instance, using Twitter (now known as X) as a means for discussing study materials (Junco et al. 2011), this usage was positively linked to academic performance.

Although consistent evidence has shown that media multitasking during academic performance can be detrimental to performance, the subjective experiences of students seem to indicate that multitasking is a necessity. For example, adolescents have reported enjoying media multitasking behavior despite their awareness of the performance costs associated with the behavior (Bardhi et al. 2010). Similarly, it has been demonstrated that individuals receive emotional rewards from media multitasking (Kononova and Chiang 2015) and particularly engage in media multitasking combinations that provide instant gratification (Baumgartner and Wiradhany 2022). Although this might be interpreted as problematic from a cognitive efficiency perspective, it might also be interpreted more positively in that adolescents can strategically use social media to take breaks from their homework in order to help them sustain their academic activity over a longer period.

Long-Term Effects on Attention and Academic Performance

It has long been argued that frequently engaging in media multitasking might lead to increased distractibility over time (e.g., Ophir et al. 2009). For example, in a seminal study, Ophir et al. (2009) showed that individuals who engaged in media multitasking more frequently were more easily distracted by irrelevant distractors than those who engaged less frequently. This study was followed by a large number of studies investigating differences in cognitive processes among heavy and light media multitaskers. Overall, meta-analyses of these studies show that these differences are rather small (Parry and le Roux 2021; Wiradhany and Nieuwenstein 2017) but point toward higher distractibility of heavy media multitaskers. Similarly, studies have shown that individuals who media multitask more frequently report having more attention problems and impulse control issues in their everyday lives (see Wiradhany and Koerts 2021 for a meta-analysis). For instance, compared with adults, children ages 6–13 years with high attention problems, as measured by items from the "inattentive presentation" dimension of the DSM-5 criteria for ADHD (American Psychiatric Association 2022), stayed on task for a shorter duration and switched more often to a different activity when performing a computerized task (Baumgartner and Sumter 2017).

However, despite evidence of these differences, it is less clear whether media multitasking caused them or whether individuals with attention problems are simply more likely to engage in media multitasking. To gain better insights on the temporal sequence and reciprocal relationship between media multitasking and attention problems, a few studies have implemented a cross-lagged panel model in which both variables are measured repeatedly over time in the same cohort (Raymaekers et al. 2020). These models allow initial conclusions about the directionality of an effect and whether two variables tend to reinforce one another. For example, if media multitasking today predicts attention problems next month, but attention problems today do not predict media multitasking next month, this would provide initial support for the idea that media multitasking caused increases in attention problems over time. A longitudinal study of 1,400 adolescents ages 11–15 years showed that those who media multitasked more often were more likely to report attention problems in their everyday lives (Baumgartner et al. 2018). However, despite this correlation, media multitasking only predicted attention problems 3 months later for early adolescents (12- to 13-year-olds) but not for older adolescents (14- to 15-year-olds). van der Schuur et al. (2020) also reported associations between media multitasking and increased distractions during academic activities and poorer school grades. Adolescents who reported more frequent multitasking during academic activities at one point in time became increasingly distracted during academic activities 3 months later. This might indicate that adolescents who are frequently using media in situations in which they need to focus find it increasingly difficult to direct their attention during school activities. However, engaging in more frequent media multitasking at one point in time did not lead to lower school grades for these adolescents at a later point in time during one school year. This might suggest that adolescents use strategies to cope with their reduced attention during schoolwork or are able to multitask strategically (e.g., not during preparation for an important exam).

Overall, existing studies in the field point toward higher distractibility among adolescents who media multitask more often, although the effects seem to be small. The long-term effects of social media use on academic performance and cognitive abilities are even less consistent. Although a plethora of research has shown that social media is frequently used among students during academic activities (Calderwood et al. 2014) and its use frequently leads to procrastination of academic tasks, whether social media use deteriorates attention in the long run is not yet established. In a review of meta-analytical evidence, Appel et al. (2020) concluded that studies on the effects of social media on academic performance explained only about 1% of the variance in school performance and only when self-reported school performance was assessed. When objective measures of school grades were considered, no effects between social media use and academic performance were found.

Implications at the Clinical and Societal Level

Overall, a small but statistically significant relationship exists between social media use or media multitasking and information processing capabilities. At a more clinical level, these relationships are unfortunately less clear. As mentioned earlier (see "Long-Term Effects on Attention and Academic Performance"), even though there appeared to be an overall association between media multitasking and ADHD (Baumgartner and Sumter 2017; Baumgartner et al. 2018; Magen 2017), the only existing longitudinal study on adolescents (Baumgartner et al. 2018) found that media multitasking led to increased ADHD-related symptoms among early adolescents (ages 12–13), but not among middle adolescents (ages 14–15). This means that even though, on average, middle adolescents with more ADHD symptoms or attention problems tend to media multitask more often, having more attention problems at one time point does not lead to more media multitasking in the future, and vice versa. Another longitudinal study on social media use and ADHD symptoms similarly showed that although, on average, individuals with a higher number of ADHD symptoms used social media more intensely and experienced more social media problems (measured using the adapted diagnostic criteria for internet gaming disorder; American Psychiatric Association 2013), having more ADHD symptoms did not lead to increased social media use in the future, and vice versa (Boer et al. 2020). Interestingly, however, a high level of problematic social media use did predict more ADHD symptoms in the future.

In sum, the limited existing evidence suggests that adolescents with ADHD are more likely to use social media and tend to media multitask more frequently. Whether, however, these phenomena reinforce one another is not yet conclusively studied. Additional research on the long-term effects of social media use and media multitasking are direly needed.

Meta-analytic estimates of media-related effects have been demonstrated to be consistently small to moderate (Valkenburg and Peter 2013). This includes effects on outcome variables that relate to cognitive processing and clinical problems such as ADHD, of which estimates range from $r=0.01$ to $r=0.12$ (Beyens et al. 2018). These small effects may curb the need to develop interventions that restrict media multitasking (Parry and le Roux 2019) or policies that restrict device use (Campbell 2006). At the same time, as Valkenburg and Peter (2013) suggested, much remains to be known regarding the boundary conditions, person- and environment-level modulators, and direction of causality of the effects of social media use or media multitasking on cognitive processing and academic performance. It could be that social media effects are especially detrimental for youth with poor levels of inhibition, namely, that youth with poor levels of self-control are more likely to access social media. This behavior would negatively impact academic performance once this becomes habitual (Fiorella 2020), and this in turn might reinforce existing low levels of self-control (Baumgartner et al. 2018; Slater 2015). With these considerations in mind, we identify two settings in which social media engagement might interfere with cognitive processing: when the engagement is triggered exogenously in the form of *disruption* or endogenously in the form of *task switching*.

Disruption and the State of Flow

Many features of social media were designed to attract attention. For instance, notification badges serve as an important visual cue for attention orienting; application (app) notifications that were accompanied by badges were more likely to be clicked (Bartoli and Benedetto 2022). Moreover, app notifications have been shown to increase habitual app use (Schnauber-Stockmann and Naab 2019). Notifications and other types of low-level visual cues might prompt youth to switch constantly from their current task to social media, or from one media to another (Brasel and Gips 2017). To complicate this matter further, young people may initiate their interactions with social media automatically in an unplanned manner, and they may continuously engage with social media unless they become aware of being distracted (Aagaard 2021). Distractions and task switching are likely to break our *state of flow*, a state in which one is fully engaged in the task at hand without much self-referential thinking, which helps us reach optimal performance (Dietrich 2004). As a result of this loss of flow, our day becomes fragmented (González and Mark 2004), and our task completion becomes less efficient due to the "awareness lag"—that is, the time it takes for us to notice that we are being distracted (Aagaard 2021)—and the "resumption lag," which is the effort we invest in reviewing where we left off in the current task once we resume it (Hausen et al. 2014). Thus, youth need to become aware of the costs of being distracted, and they may want to structure their environment to limit distractions (Fiorella 2020), such as by installing apps that prevent or limit social media access or by turning off notifications on distracting apps (Aagaard 2021).

The long-term impact of constant media multitasking behavior still needs to be investigated. Although some initial longitudinal studies found only limited evidence for long-term effects of media multitasking on attention and academic distractibility (e.g., van der Schuur et al. 2020), other studies found that media multitasking is associated with increased stress (Bardhi et al. 2010; Mark et al. 2014). From the perspective of attention systems, each additional medium we consume during a given time window contributes to the gross changes in our tonic alertness, of which overactivity might cause distress that has an adverse impact on learning (Teigen 1994). Stress limits vary from one youth to another, and because youth is a life period during which many stressors appear (Arnett 1999), young people need to become increasingly aware of when and under which conditions social media–related distractions offer much-needed breaks that prevent boredom and under which conditions such diversions are experienced as stressful and distract from the tasks at hand.

Optimal Switching and Wakeful Rest

The abundance of social media in our everyday situations presents us with a constant dilemma: should I abandon the task at hand, or inhibit the need to check social media? We call this the *exploration-exploitation dilemma* (Wiradhany et al. 2021). Continuing with the task at hand constitutes an *exploitation*; it has a clear goal and known reward. Checking the notification constitutes an *exploration*; it leads us away from the current goal but has the potential to provide a reward. How long should we "exploit" a task before we start "exploring" other options in our environment? Although we might expect persistent exploitation to be the most optimal behavior, it has been shown that exploring in between might also be beneficial. For example, intermittent active breaks, such as walking or stretching, had beneficial impacts on work productivity (Bosch and Sonnentag 2018) and learning (Howie et al. 2015).

Initial studies have shown that people switch from one task to another adaptively at their "natural breaking points." For instance, in a simulation study in which participants switched from answering emails and instant messages, Salvucci and Bogunovich (2010) found that most task switches occurred during low-workload periods. Thus, particularly during adolescence, it might be important to train these abilities in order to multitask more adaptively. Future studies might consider to what extent individual differences in sensation-seeking (Dalley et al. 2011), self-regulation, and polychronicity (i.e., one's propensity toward multitasking) (König and Waller 2010) contribute to this phenomenon.

Youth might access social media during breaks (Calderwood et al. 2014; Martini et al. 2020) as a means to replenish their mental resources. From the attention systems perspective, checking social media might provide a "mini-task" that could be completed without much attentional resources (Szumowska and Kossowska 2017). However, social media engagement also might backfire; one recent study showed that spending 8 minutes posting, liking, and commenting on Facebook and Instagram as opposed to taking a wakeful rest (laying one's head on one's arms, closing one's eyes, and resting quietly) had a negative impact on immediate and delayed memory recall performance on a vocabulary test (Martini et al. 2020). Future studies might investigate further to what extent accessing social media, compared with taking other types of breaks, contributes to changes in cognitive and affective states.

Conclusion

Our cognitive systems naturally modulate, (re)orient, and control attention in everyday situations. The proliferation of social media over recent years has arguably overburdened our cognitive systems and impedes effective information processing. Our review of the current literature suggests that, although there is consistent evidence for the negative impact of social media and media multitasking on information processing and academic performance, the magnitude of the effects is small. Because much is yet unknown about individual susceptibilities and boundary conditions in these effects, it may be too soon to create concrete policies or interventions that restrict social media use. At the same time, further investigations are needed to determine the boundary conditions, person- and environment-level modulators, and direction of causality regarding the association between social media use/media multitasking and cognitive processing/academic performance. The highly rewarding and distracting nature of social media might make it increasingly difficult for young people to gain a state of flow; therefore, clinicians and educators are advised to help young people find an optimal balance between workflow and taking restful breaks. In addition, we need a clearer understanding of interventions and tools that might help those adolescents who are particularly prone to digital distractions (e.g., those showing ADHD symptoms and those with impulse control difficulties).

References

Aagaard J: "From a small click to an entire action": exploring students' anti-distraction strategies. Learn Media Technol 46(3):355–365, 2021

American Psychiatric Association: Diagnostic and Statistical Manual of Mental Disorders, 5th Edition. Arlington, VA, American Psychiatric Association, 2013

American Psychiatric Association: Diagnostic and Statistical Manual of Mental Disorders, 5th Edition, Text Revision. Washington, DC, American Psychiatric Association, 2022

Appel M, Marker C, Gnambs T: Are social media ruining our lives? A review of meta-analytic evidence. Rev Gen Psychol 24(1):60–74, 2020

Arnett JJ: Adolescent storm and stress, reconsidered. Am Psychol 54(5):317–326, 1999 10354802

Aston-Jones G, Cohen JD: An integrative theory of locus coeruleus-norepinephrine function: adaptive gain and optimal performance. Annu Rev Neurosci 28(1):403–450, 2005 16022602

Bardhi F, Rohm AJ, Sultan F: Tuning in and tuning out: media multitasking among young consumers. J Consum Behav 9:316–332, 2010

Bartoli N, Benedetto S: Driven by notifications: exploring the effects of badge notifications on user experience. PLoS One 17(6):e0270888, 2022

Baumgartner SE, Sumter SR: Dealing with media distractions: an observational study of computer-based multitasking among children and adults in the Netherlands. J Child Media 11(3):295–313, 2017

Baumgartner SE, Wiradhany W: Not all media multitasking is the same: the frequency of media multitasking depends on cognitive and affective characteristics of media combinations. Psychol Pop Media 11(1):1–12, 2022

Baumgartner SE, van der Schuur WA, Lemmens JS, et al: The relationship between media multitasking and attention problems in adolescents: results of two longitudinal studies. Hum Commun Res 44(1):3–30, 2018

Bayer JB, Triệu P, Ellison NB: Social media elements, ecologies, and effects. Annu Rev Psychol 71(1):471–497, 2020 31518525

Beyens I, Valkenburg PM, Piotrowski JT: Screen media use and ADHD-related behaviors: four decades of research. Proc Natl Acad Sci U S A 115(40):9875–9881, 2018 30275318

Boer M, Stevens G, Finkenauer C, et al: Attention deficit hyperactivity disorder—symptoms, social media use intensity, and social media use problems in adolescents: investigating directionality. Child Dev 91(4):e853–e865, 2020 31654398

Bosch C, Sonnentag S: Should I take a break? A daily reconstruction study on predicting micro-breaks at work. Int J Stress Manag 26(4):378–388, 2018

Botvinick M, Braver T: Motivation and cognitive control: from behavior to neural mechanism. Annu Rev Psychol 66(1):83–113, 2015 25251491

Brasel SA, Gips J: Media multitasking behavior: concurrent television and computer usage. Cyberpsychol Behav Soc Netw 14(9):527–534, 2011 21381969

Brasel SA, Gips J: Media multitasking: how visual cues affect switching behavior. Comput Human Behav 77:258–265, 2017

Brooks S: Does personal social media usage affect efficiency and well-being? Comput Human Behav 46:26–37, 2015

Calderwood C, Ackerman PL, Conklin EM: What else do college students "do" while studying? An investigation of multitasking. Comput Educ 75:19–29, 2014

Campbell SW: Perceptions of mobile phones in college classrooms: ringing, cheating, and classroom policies. Commun Educ 55(3):280–294, 2006

Corbetta M, Patel G, Shulman GL: The reorienting system of the human brain: from environment to theory of mind. Neuron 58(3):306–324, 2008 18466742

Dalley JW, Everitt BJ, Robbins TW: Impulsivity, compulsivity, and top-down cognitive control. Neuron 69(4):680–694, 2011 21338879

Dietrich A: Neurocognitive mechanisms underlying the experience of flow. Conscious Cogn 13(4):746–761, 2004 15522630

Downs E, Tran A, McMenemy R, et al: Exam performance and attitudes toward multitasking in six, multimedia-multitasking classroom environments. Comput Educ 86:250–259, 2015

Fan J, McCandliss BD, Sommer T, et al: Testing the efficiency and independence of attentional networks. J Cogn Neurosci 14(3):340–347, 2002 11970796

Fan J, McCandliss BD, Fossella J, et al: The activation of attentional networks. Neuroimage 26(2):471–479, 2005 15907304

Fiorella L: The science of habit and its implications for student learning and well-being. Educ Psychol Rev 32:603–625, 2020

González VM, Mark G: "Constant, constant, multi-tasking craziness": managing multiple working spheres. Presented at the Proceedings of the 2004 Conference on Human Factors in Computing Systems, CHI 2004, Vienna, Austria, April 24–29, 2004

Hausen D, Loehmann S, Lehmann M: Everyday peripheral tasks vs. digital peripheral tasks, in CHI'14 Extended Abstracts on Human Factors in Computing Systems. New York, Association for Computing Machinery, 2014, pp 2545–2550

Howie EK, Schatz J, Pate RR: Acute effects of classroom exercise breaks on executive function and math performance: a dose-response study. Res Q Exerc Sport 86(3):217–224, 2015 26009945

Junco R, Heiberger G, Loken E: The effect of Twitter on college student engagement and grades. J Comput Assist Learn 27(2):119–132, 2011

König CJ, Waller MJ: Time for reflection: a critical examination of polychronicity. Hum Perform 23(2):173–190, 2010

Kononova A, Chiang Y-H: Why do we multitask with media? Predictors of media multitasking among internet users in the United States and Taiwan. Comput Human Behav 50:31–41, 2015

Lin L: Breadth-biased versus focused cognitive control in media multitasking behaviors. Proc Natl Acad Sci USA 106(37):15521–15522, 2009 19805207

Magen H: The relations between executive functions, media multitasking and polychronicity. Comput Human Behav 67:1–9, 2017

Mahoney JR, Verghese J, Goldin Y, et al: Alerting, orienting, and executive attention in older adults. J Int Neuropsychol Soc 16(5):877–889, 2010 20663241

Mark G, Wang Y, Niiya M: Stress and multitasking in everyday college life, in CHI'14 Extended Abstracts on Human Factors in Computing Systems. New York, Association for Computing Machinery, 2014, pp 41–50

Marker C, Gnambs T, Appel M: Active on Facebook and failing at school? Meta-analytic findings on the relationship between online social networking activities and academic achievement. Educ Psychol Rev 30(3):651–677, 2018

Martini M, Heinz A, Hinterholzer J, et al: Effects of wakeful resting versus social media usage after learning on the retention of new memories. Appl Cogn Psychol 34(2):551–558, 2020

Mezzacappa E: Alerting, orienting, and executive attention: developmental properties and sociodemographic correlates in an epidemiological sample of young, urban children. Child Dev 75(5):1373–1386, 2004 15369520

Mullane JC, Lawrence MA, Corkum PV, et al: The development of and interaction among alerting, orienting, and executive attention in children. Child Neuropsychol 22(2):155–176, 2016 25413609

Ophir E, Nass C, Wagner AD: Cognitive control in media multitaskers. Proc Natl Acad Sci USA 106(37):15583–15587, 2009 19706386

Parry DA, le Roux DB: Media multitasking and cognitive control: a systematic review of interventions. Comput Human Behav 92:316–327, 2019

Parry DA, le Roux DB: "Cognitive control in media multitaskers" ten years on: a meta-analysis. Cyberpsychology (Brno) 15(2):Article 7, 2021

Petersen SE, Posner MI: The attention system of the human brain: 20 years after. Annu Rev Neurosci 35(1):73–89, 2012 22524787

Posner MI, Petersen SE: The attention system of the human brain. Annu Rev Neurosci 13:25–42, 1990 2183676

Raymaekers K, Luyckx K, Moons P: A guide to improve your causal inferences from observational data. Eur J Cardiovasc Nurs 19(8):757–762, 2020 33040589

Rothbart MK, Rueda MR: The development of effortful control, in Developing Individuality in the Human Brain: A Tribute to Michael I. Posner. Edited by Mayr U, Keele S. Washington, DC, American Psychological Association, 2005, pp 167–188

Salvucci DD, Bogunovich P: Multitasking and monotasking: the effects of mental workload on deferred task interruptions, in Extended Abstracts on Human Factors in Computing Systems. New York, Association for Computing Machinery, 2010, pp 85–88

Schnauber-Stockmann A, Naab TK: The process of forming a mobile media habit: results of a longitudinal study in a real-world setting. Media Psychol 22(5):714–742, 2019

Segijn CM, Voorveld HAM, Vandeberg L, et al: The battle of the screens: unraveling attention allocation and memory effects when multiscreening. Hum Commun Res 43(2):295–314, 2017

Slater MD: Reinforcing spirals model: conceptualizing the relationship between media content exposure and the development and maintenance of attitudes. Media Psychol 18(3):370–395, 2015 26366124

Szumowska E, Kossowska M: Motivational rigidity enhances multitasking performance: the role of handling interruptions. Pers Individ Dif 106:81–89, 2017

Szumowska E, Kruglanski AW: The psychology of getting busy: multitasking as a consequence of goal activation. J Exp Psychol Gen 151(1):137–160, 2022 35238599

Teigen KH: Yerkes-Dodson: a law for all seasons. Theory Psychol 4(4):525–547, 1994

Uncapher MR, Lin L, Rosen LD, et al: Media multitasking and cognitive, psychological, neural, and learning differences. Pediatrics 140(November Suppl 2):S62–S66, 2017 29093034

Valkenburg PM, Peter J: The differential susceptibility to media effects model. J Commun 63(2):221–243, 2013

van der Schuur WA, Baumgartner SE, Sumter SR, et al: Exploring the long-term relationship between academic-media multitasking and adolescents' academic achievement. New Media Soc 22(1):140–158, 2020

Vogels EA, Gelles-Watnick R, Massarat N: Teens, social media and technology 2022. Pew Research Center, August 10, 2022. Available at: https://www.pewresearch.org/internet/2022/08/10/teens-social-media-and-technology-2022. Accessed December 2, 2023.

Vorderer P, Hefner D, Reinecke L, et al: Permanently online, permanently connected: a new paradigm in communication research? in Permanently Online, Permanently Connected: Living and Communicating in a POPC World. Edited by Vorderer P, Hefner D, Reinecke L, et al. New York, Routledge, 2018

Wiradhany W, Koerts J: Everyday functioning-related cognitive correlates of media multitasking: a mini meta-analysis. Media Psychol 24(2):276–303, 2021

Wiradhany W, Nieuwenstein MR: Cognitive control in media multitaskers: two replication studies and a meta-analysis. Atten Percept Psychophys 79(8):2620–2641, 2017 28840547

Wiradhany W, Baumgartner SE, de Bruin ABH: Exploitation: exploration model of media multitasking. J Media Psychol 33(4):169–180, 2021

Yu AJ, Dayan P: Uncertainty, neuromodulation, and attention. Neuron 46(4):681–692, 2005 15944135

10

Intersectional Identities Online

Race, Gender, Culture, Sex, Class

Cătălina Maria Popoviciu, M.A.

Intersectionality is a term that Kimberley Crenshaw (1989) coined "to speak to the multiple social forces, social identities, and ideological instruments through which power and disadvantage are expressed and legitimized." It means that individuals experience discrimination and privilege based on the intersection of their various identities—such as race, sex/gender, sexual orientation, class, and socioeconomic status. Because intersectionality recognizes that people can experience multiple forms of oppression simultaneously and that these experiences cannot be fully understood by looking at any one identity in isolation, it is a crucial framework for understanding how power and inequality operate online for individuals of all ages. In this chapter, I use the intersectionality framework to provide insights into social media's potential benefits and harms for young people's mental health and well-being.

I would like to express my sincere gratitude to Dr. Allison Briscoe-Smith for her valuable feedback and support throughout the writing process. Her expertise and insights were invaluable in shaping the chapter.

Where youth are concerned, the intersectionality theory highlights the importance of the interaction among the multiple facets of their identities for their mental health and in shaping well-being outcomes. The theory focuses on seeing the individual as a whole, but with complex identity dimensions. The term *identity* is defined in this chapter through the lens of the social identity theory, which refers to the different ways people categorize themselves and others based on social characteristics or group memberships (Abrams and Hogg 1990); these identities can include, but are not limited to, race, sex/gender, sexuality, age, religion, nationality, socioeconomic status, and other axes of social power. The *intersectionality* term has been used widely in the social sciences to understand the offline experiences of marginalized groups (Collins and Bilge 2020; Crenshaw 2017; de Vries 2012). However, when it comes to the social media world, evidence of applying the theory is scarce.

> Most of the time, I feel as though discrimination or insensitive jokes target a specific part of my identities (Asian ching chong jokes, Dutch weed jokes) and never the entirety. If they did see the entirety of my identity or looked deep enough, I imagine for a lot of people empathy would kick in somehow. It's that superficiality and willful ignorance that keeps any kind of "damn this person is kind of like me" at bay.
>
> —*Dion, Netherlands, age 22*

Social media has become an increasingly important part of young people's lives and has transformed the way youth interact and present themselves to the world, evolving as well into a platform in which their various social identities intersect, providing a unique opportunity for both empowerment and marginalization. Social media provides spaces for intersectional identities to be expressed and celebrated and can help youth to connect, explore their personalities and creativity, find community, and receive peer support, but it can also be an oppressive environment with negative consequences for their mental health and well-being. Social media can perpetuate stereotypes about race, class, and sex/gender; reinforce discrimination, biases, cyberbullying, and harassment; be a fruitful landscape where oppressive constructs emerge and are reinforced; and have far-reaching mental health implications such as social comparison, self-image and body image issues, substance use, depression, anxiety, social isolation, and suicide risk

(Alhajji et al. 2019; Hinduja and Patchin 2008; Keum and Cano 2021; Patchin and Hinduja 2006; Perloff 2014). For instance, youth who are Black, Indigenous, and people of color (BIPOC) may face online harassment and hate speech specifically rooted in racism (Francisco and Felmlee 2022). Similarly, youth who identify as women or as members of the LGBTQ+ community may face harassment and discrimination based on their gender or sexual orientation (Cote 2017; Uttarapong et al. 2021). Black women who are part of the LGBTQ+ community may face even higher marginalization based on expressing their multiple identities (Brown 2021; Uttarapong et al. 2021). Youth from low-income backgrounds may face barriers to accessing the internet and participating fully in online spaces, leading to a digital divide (Eamon 2004).

> On the internet, people hold widely different views about the Asian part of my ethnicity. Sometimes they share these beliefs in a manner that bothers me, through assumptions about my competency in maths or assumptions about me being socially inept because I "study all day." Most of the time, however, the line between discrimination and "preference" blurs. It is hard to criticize behaviors that find themselves on both ends of that spectrum.
>
> —*Dion, Netherlands, age 22*

Users bring their racial identities online, as well as their class, sex/gender, sexual orientation, and religion, among other embodied identities and experiences. The intersection of these identities then shapes the user's interactions in the online world and may affect their contribution to a wider conversation. These online interactions offer the potential for both challenging and reinforcing norms and behaviors and for individuals' intersectional perspectives on various subjects to either support or undermine the ideological foundations of a movement. The impact of these interactions can be felt on both personal and societal levels (Noble and Tynes 2016). For instance, a person who identifies as a Black woman brings her intersectional identity into an online conversation about feminism along with her perspectives on gender equality, which may be informed by her experiences with racism and sexism and may differ from the perspectives of White feminists. In this context, her contributions to the conversation may challenge the dominant narrative and bring attention to the experiences of women of color. If her views are dismissed or marginalized by other participants in the conversation, it can reinforce existing power imbalances and undermine the primary goal of the movement.

Social Media and Identity

> I think social media has a lot of advantages in terms of identity—you can meet others who share your traits, and I have found it particularly helpful in finding community and feeling less alone in certain aspects of my identity.
> —*Anna, United Kingdom, 26 years old*

Social and psychological identity formation is a vital stage of adolescence (Erikson 1968; McAdams 2015), which is a period marked by major changes in biology, cognitive functioning, and social interactions (Bell 2016) and is a prolonged phase referred to in modern culture as *emerging adulthood* (Arnett et al. 2014). Developing the capacity to construct and maintain a feeling of personal continuity through time and across diverse situations is an important element of both psychological and social identity formation during this period (Erikson 1968; Pasupathi et al. 2007). Adolescents must determine how to succeed in friendships with their peers, exercise their social duties as appropriate, and pick from numerous views, ideas, and possibilities that will provide them with a feeling of separate and autonomous life as they work to establish their own destiny (National Academies of Sciences, Engineering, and Medicine et al. 2019).

The online environment plays a crucial role in this developmental phase and significantly influences how young people view and exhibit themselves to others. Social media allows youth to explore different aspects of their personality; showcase their values, thoughts, and beliefs; express themselves in ways that were previously not possible; connect with others who share similar interests and experiences; and find acceptance and validation from their peers (Allen et al. 2014; Bozzola et al. 2022).

Some evidence on social media and identity suggests that online and offline identities may overlap to a certain degree (Coleman 2011), whereas other evidence proposes that youth experience a "networked self" in which identity is constructed through online interactions and communities (Buckingham 2007). Anonymity in the online world allows youth to create different personas and idealized selves that can differ from their offline self. They can also add values to their online identity that they think are missing from their offline self (Qin and Lowe 2021). Social media may contribute to the creation, construction, and reconstruction of the psychological and social identity (Huang et al. 2021). In addition, the feedback youth receive on social media can have a major impact on their identity formation; positive feedback received through likes, comments, or shares can boost self-esteem and confidence, reinforce youth's beliefs and values, and perhaps help them choose a peer-support community of interest (Metzler and Scheithauer 2017). Social media can be an important tool for youth to explore and affirm their gender and sexual identities (Berger et al. 2022) and can represent a space to connect with others who share their cultural or ethnic identities, which can be especially important for youth from marginalized communities (Evans 2022).

> It would be amazing to include your identity on the sign-up page so the platforms could recommend accounts with the same identities. This could bring users into a community they never knew about.
> —*Anna, United Kingdom, age 26*

However, this new unregulated terrain can be detrimental to young people's development of identity, particularly for those who belong to marginalized groups (Matamoros-Fernández and Farkas 2021; Schemer et al. 2021). Social media is not a neutral arena any more than any offline space. Here, too, the experiences of young people are affected by their many aspects of identity, such as race, sex/gender, culture, and class (Noble and Tynes 2016). For instance, an LGBTQ+ youth from a rural area can find community and support from their peers but face discrimination and harmful stereotypes that, in turn, might have an impact on their identity formation and views about themselves. Digital media also provides new avenues for monitoring and control and can exercise power in both subtle and overt ways. With private companies tracking user data and algorithmically providing information and government authorities censoring information and media content (Gillespie 2018; Stieglitz and Dang-Xuan 2013), the online space can curtail youth self-expression and limit the diversity of information and perspectives available to them. These restrictions can have an overall chilling effect on online dialogue and creativity that will ultimately lead to a lack of agency for youth over their identity, impede their personal development and their ability to build meaningful relationships with others, and affect their well-being.

Intersectionality is a critical lens for understanding the complex and multifaceted ways in which an individual's different identity factors intersect and form experiences in online spaces, as well as how these experiences affect youth mental health and well-being.

Algorithms, Search Engines, and Oppressive Constructs Online

> Social media platforms have to make an effort on how they filter the content because their censorship policy is blocking posts that are not supposed to be censored.
>
> —*Malia, Portugal, age 22*

The algorithms used by social media companies can perpetuate biases and discrimination by favoring and amplifying content created by individuals with more privilege while suppressing or marginalizing content created by disadvantaged groups (Noble 2018; Roberts 2019). These biases can create a feedback loop in which people with more privilege are seen and heard while those with less privilege are silenced and excluded. The algorithms can also reinforce the *echo chamber effect* phenomenon, in which users are only exposed to information and perspectives that align with their preexisting beliefs, further solidifying harmful attitudes and behaviors in some cases (Cinelli et al. 2021) and posing a threat to young people from marginalized communities. A study of 15 TikTok users demonstrated that the social media algorithm may actively suppress content related to marginalized social identities, proposing "The Identity Strainer Theory" as a way to describe the algorithmic social media suppression faced by marginalized communities (Karizat et al. 2021). As Noble (2018) stated, the design of the algorithms and recommendation engines reflects the biases of their creators and the societies in which they operate, creating the perfect platform for oppressive constructs to emerge. The power of social media algorithms is reinforced in the literature by what Noble coined as *technological redlining*, explaining that the algorithms, while ostensibly objective and fair, are in fact biased toward particular demographics and further reinforce existing structures of inequality. Technological redlining, as a form of discrimination and bias, can have severe consequences for marginalized communities, particularly with regard to access to education, health care, and employment opportunities (Noble 2018).

One study found that Facebook's ad-targeting algorithm allowed advertisers to discriminate against job seekers based on age, sex/gender, and race by promoting roles to only certain users (Imana et al. 2021). The study revealed that certain job postings still display a significant bias, even when the job requirements are identical to jobs that reflect real-world sex/gender demographics. Another online survey on Twitter's binary treatment of gender, which sought to identify whether gender inferences by Twitter algorithms contained inaccuracies, revealed that its algorithms misgendered users in nearly 20% of the cases, and only 8% of the straight male respondents were misgendered compared with 25% of gay males and 16% of straight females (Fosch-Villaronga et al. 2021). Twitter (known as X since 2023) uses multiple sources, such as account information, link interactions, and cookie data, to determine users' identity but not their sexual orientation.

Furthermore, it has been observed that social media algorithms censor content shared by marginalized communities by banning key phrases or words (Lorenz 2022). Members of the LGBTQ+ or BIPOC communities are "timed out" (e.g., having their posts removed or down-ranked) from social media platforms if they use the banned phrases, leading to the rise of "algospeak" slang on social media platforms (e.g., using the phrase "leg booty" for LGBTQ issues, "AI Gore" for algorithms, and "le$bian" instead of lesbian) to avoid algorithmic detection and deletion. When youth are talking about mental health issues, they say they are talking about "becoming unalive" in order to openly be able to talk about suicide or depression without being censored by the platform (Lorenz 2022). This type of treatment happens across platforms. The banning of certain words or phrases is not necessarily an intentional form of oppression but, rather, a means to enforce community standards and promote user safety (e.g., minimizing harmful content such as the pro-suicide material). However, this unintended consequence can lead to the censorship of important conversations and information sharing, particularly within marginalized communities, impeding their ability to find the support they need and to connect with others.

Social media algorithms may create "bubbles" based on young people's online data, formed through browsing history, likes and follows, demographic data, or data tracked from other websites. These bubbles may expose youth from marginalized communities to stigmatizing and harmful reinforced content or to content in which youth are underrepresented, which can further exacerbate existing inequalities and discrimination. The bubbles also shield young people from new experiences and perspectives.

Moreover, Buolamwini and Gebru (2018) conducted a study that evaluated the gender classification accuracy of three commercial Application Programming Interface (API)-based classifiers using facial images. The study revealed that the classifiers' recognition abilities were not equally distributed across genders and skin tones. Using facial recognition technology, the researchers identified gender classification discrepancies: dark-skinned women had the highest error rate compared with light-skinned men, who experienced more accurate results. Equally important, Noble (2018) argued that search engines, particularly Google, reinforce and perpetuate societal biases and discrimination through their algorithms and the way they rank and display search results. For instance, search results for the word *beautiful* are dominated by images of White females, which can perpetuate the harmful idea that beauty is primarily White and Eurocentric, consequently perpetuating a lack of visibility and representation for people of color and other marginalized groups.

Algorithms demonstrate how digital technologies can not only "digitalize oppression" but also reshape structural oppression based on race, sex/gender, and sexuality, as well as identities' intersectional relationships and their impact on mental health. Although algorithms and search engines may appear to be complex, they are simply pieces of code written and developed by humans who have their own biases (Bivens and Haimson 2016; Noble 2018; Noble and Tynes 2016). As stated earlier in this section, algorithms are not neutral entities but rather reflect the biases and values of their creators; they can perpetuate existing power dynamics and reinforce societal inequalities. This emphasizes the need for more diverse representation and perspectives in the technology industry to ensure that algorithms are developed and implemented more inclusively and equitably.

Online Experiences for Youth With Intersectional Identities

Online Harassment and Hate Speech

I have been bullied by classmates, physically threatened and harassed by strangers on the street/public transport to the point of having to call authorities in that instance, and experiencing a panic attack the next time I went on public transport. I have been called racist remarks ceaselessly, and by both men and women. People have imitated "ching-chong eyes," staring me down and throwing fake-out punches at me. People have started speaking in gibberish

Chinese/Japanese to me. On social media, it should arguably be easier to engage in behaviors like these because I
wouldn't be able to call authorities or retaliate, but again, I
can be selective with who I engage with. I can block. I can
only add people I like. I can delete followers. I can make my
profile private. All of these options are at my disposal and
make me feel safer.

—Dion, Netherlands, age 22

A Pew Research Center survey conducted in 2022 found that nearly half of
U.S. teens ages 13–17 (46%) have experienced cyberbullying, while other
studies showed that most 18- to 29-year-olds (65%) have experienced some
form of hate or harassment, with 49% reporting severe harassment (Vogels
2022). YouTube banned 85,247 videos for hate speech violations from January to March 2021, while Facebook took action against 25.2 million pieces
of such content and Instagram against 6.3 million during the same period.
In the second half of 2020, Twitter found 1,628,281 items in breach of its hate
speech policy (UNESCO 2021).

Research suggests that one-third of online harassment and hate speech
may be motivated by the target's protected characteristics, such as race or
ethnicity, religion, gender identity, sexual orientation, or disability (Anti-
Defamation League 2019; Obermaier 2022). LGBTQ+, Muslim, Hispanic,
and Black people face disproportionately high levels of identity-based discrimination (Anti-Defamation League 2019), with some studies showing
that pansexual and bisexual youth report extensively more negative experiences of harassment and exclusion across all major social media platforms
compared with their lesbian and gay peers (Nelson et al. 2023). Online harassment and cyberbullying are a significant concern for youth of all genders, races, classes, and cultures.

Young people from marginalized groups face more negativity and harassment online (Vogels 2022) than their peers. They are more likely to self-
censor their posts to avoid it and may feel less inclined to speak out against
injustice or to share their experiences, which can help reinforce oppressive
constructs online. For instance, a study examined the online habits and race-
related experiences of 264 school students ages 14–18 years, revealing that
71% of Black, 71% of White, and 67% of multiracial/other adolescents reported vicarious racial discrimination online (Tynes et al. 2008).

Compared with males, females are more than twice as likely to report being sexually harassed online and are more vulnerable to physical threats and

sustained harassment. Tynes and Mitchell (2014) examined Black youth's online behaviors and victimization experiences using a subsample of Black adolescents, with findings suggesting that young Black females were more likely than young Black males to report encountering individuals online who threatened, harassed, or bothered them. Recent evidence on Twitter/X showed that one emerging theme in tweets targeting Black females was accusations of promiscuity, with messages including slurs accusing them of being overly sexual (Francisco and Felmlee 2022). Xenophobia was a recurring topic in messages containing Latinx slurs, with common terms related to menial labor and political comments invoking the need to "build a wall." Appearance-related insults were also directed at both groups of females (Francisco and Felmlee 2022).

A recent report from GLAAD's 2022 Social Media Safety Index, which utilized 12 LGBTQ+-specific indicators in order to generate numeric ratings for LGBTQ+ safety, privacy, and expression on social media platforms, showed that all platforms scored below 50 out of a possible 100 (GLAAD 2022). Black LGBTQ+ youth are at higher risk for online harassment, with studies showing that they experience higher rates of cyberbullying compared with their non-Black and non-LGBTQ+ peers (Alhajji et al. 2019). The intersection of their identities as Black and LGBTQ+ leads to a unique and synergistic experience of online harassment, with participants reporting that they have been targeted with racist and homophobic language.

> Just being a woman is enough to get some forms of harassment on social media, like microaggressions.
> —*anonymous, Romania, age 24*

Online harassment reflects the systemic racial discrimination and gendered power relations that characterize contemporary women's experiences. Digital technologies, and specifically social media, amplify gender and race-based attacks. An example of a high-profile case of online harassment is that experienced by tennis player Serena Williams, who endured a significant amount of abuse on social media during the 2015 Wimbledon tournament (Litchfield et al. 2018). This case highlights issues of gender, race, and identity as enacted through social media and the impact of online harassment on individuals. As Litchfield et al. (2018) discussed in their study, "Williams identifies as female and African American, so intersectionality was used to examine her representation in social media spaces." Their case analysis brought to light several topics relating to Williams, including gender questioning, accusations of performance-enhancing drug use, and racism, which "demonstrated the overlapping of multiple forms of oppression Williams experienced, reinforcing the notion of the Black female athlete as the 'other' in virtual spaces." The authors note that online environments exacerbate such oppression (Litchfield et al. 2018).

Research has shown that online harassment can have a severe impact on youth mental health and well-being, particularly for minorities (Alhajji et al. 2019), placing victims at greater risk for emotional distress, absenteeism, substance use, suicidal behavior, and even PTSD (Abreu and Kenny 2017; Hawton and Stewart 2018; Mateu et al. 2020; Maurya et al. 2022; Selkie et al. 2015; Zhu et al. 2021). Studies show that victims of online harassment may lack appropriate coping strategies to mitigate the harm and are less likely to report and seek help than those affected by offline harassment (Kaiser et al. 2020).

Social Media as a Supportive Environment

Despite these problems, social media presents positives as well. It can provide a valuable platform for marginalized communities and youth to connect, share information, raise awareness, and act on issues that matter to them. It can empower them to have their voices heard and to advocate for change in their communities. This can lead to the formation of online support groups and the sharing of resources and information, which can help counteract feelings of isolation and marginalization that they may experience offline. Additionally, social media can provide opportunities for youth to express themselves and their identities in a safe and supportive environment—they can build communities, develop their social skills, and gain a sense of empowerment, belonging, and agency (Buckingham 2007). Social media can be a powerful tool to break down barriers and foster dialogue between youth and other members of their communities.

I think [social media] is the most powerful tool nowadays because it incorporates so many features that can help create posts for the purpose of informing [a] mass of people about different communities, not just with texts but also images. Moreover, I think [it's possible to] ask about the experiences of people with intersectional identities, about their difficulties, and to take action based on their answers.
—*anonymous, Romania, age 24*

Through social media, young people can engage in conversations and dialogue about a wide range of topics, from mental health and well-being to social justice and civic engagement. Hashtags used on social media allow individuals to find and join conversations about specific topics, and they can be particularly useful for marginalized communities who lack visibility or representation within mainstream media. For example, the hashtag #BlackLivesMatter has been used to bring attention to issues of racial injustice and police brutality and has helped mobilize and organize protests and other forms of civic engagement (Black Lives Matter 2021). Similarly, hashtags such as #TransRightsAreHumanRights (Instagram; www.instagram.com/explore/tags/transrightsarehumanrights/?hl=af) and #DisabledAndProud (TikTok; www.tiktok.com/tag/disabledandproud) can help raise awareness of issues facing trans and disabled communities, respectively, and provide a platform for members of these communities to share their experiences and advocate for their rights. As noted by Olayinka et al. (2021), the hashtag #BlackGirlMagic, developed in response to a now-deleted article posted in *Psychology Today* that stated Black women were "objectively less physically attractive than other women," sparked a nationwide empowerment movement that served to celebrate Black women's achievements while affirming their beauty in a world that rarely does so.

Social media also can provide a platform for young people to engage in activism and civic engagement by using hashtags and creating their own campaigns to raise awareness and advocate for change. This may have a significant impact on the visibility and representation of marginalized communities in society because their stories are being told in a more accessible manner. These campaigns can be used to educate others about the experiences and perspectives of marginalized communities and to advocate for policies and practices that will benefit these communities. Such campaigns can also help bridge the gap between privileged and marginalized communities by bringing people together through a shared understanding of the issues and their importance. For instance, the #SayHerName campaign uses hashtags and reposts to spread the word about injustices against Black females (Brown et al. 2017), and the #MyIdentity campaign, launched on Instagram and Twitter in 2018 by a group of young people from New Zealand, is an example of a youth-led campaign about intersectional identities online (New Zealand Herald 2018). Young people from various marginalized communities use this hashtag to raise awareness about the experiences of and unique challenges faced by individuals with multiple marginalized identities by sharing their personal stories and experiences under different categories such as race, sex/gender, religion, sexual orientation, and so on. The campaign educates others about intersectionality and the importance of understanding the unique experiences of individuals with multiple marginalized identities, helping to create a more inclusive online community and encouraging others to be more mindful of the ways in which different forms of oppression intersect and affect different individuals in different ways (New Zealand Herald 2018).

> 100%, I had positive events with social media, around events like Pride, and [mental health] awareness week. It has been lovely to see others share their experiences and bring positivity to the platform. I do find seeing other people living their identities very comforting as it feels like a shared experience.
> —*Bailie, United Kingdom, age 26*

Social media can provide a safe space for youth to connect with others who share similar experiences and to express themselves freely. These connections can improve mental health by providing a sense of understanding, acceptance, and community. For example, youth who identify as LGBTQ+ may not feel comfortable expressing their sexual orientation or gender identity in their offline communities due to societal prejudices and discrimination, and the online world could be a safe environment to find support (Andalibi et al. 2022). Other studies suggest that young Black females who used social media were more likely to report higher levels of self-esteem and a greater sense of community than their non-Black counterparts (Olayinka et al. 2021).

Conclusion and Recommendations

> In an ideal world, we would have heightened safety for all users on the platform. I worry that sometimes safety measures can further exclude people with intersectional identities, as sometimes content gets taken down [inaccurately].
> —*Bailie, United Kingdom, age 26*

As both Noble (2018) and Roberts (2019) emphasized, social media can be a double-edged sword for people with marginalized intersectional identities. The dichotomy between using technology as a tool for agency and using it as a tool for oppression is important to consider when discussing the effects of social media on marginalized individuals. In order to create a more inclusive and equitable social media landscape, it is crucial that we actively work toward dismantling the biases and discrimination built into these platforms and elevate the voices and perspectives of marginalized communities.

Some possible ways to address the issues of bias and discrimination on social media at the societal level are:

1. To develop more diverse and representative teams of engineers and designers who are responsible for creating and maintaining the platforms, offering a smooth and safe experience for the young users;
2. To actively invest in creating more diverse and representative content on social media by users, advertising companies, and social media platforms (World Advertising Research Center 2023);
3. To amplify the voices of marginalized communities and support their efforts to create and share their own narratives, such as by providing opportunities for youth and groups to speak, write, create art, and share their experiences with a wider audience through various social media platforms, providing the resources and technical assistance to tell their stories in a safe manner, and investing in digital media initiatives that promote their voices and perspectives through funding opportunities, mentorship, and resources;
4. To focus on increasing transparency and accountability around the algorithms and moderation practices used on social media platforms (Swart 2021); and
5. To establish independent oversight bodies to monitor the algorithms and moderation practices.

As for social media platforms, they should 1) disclose more information about their algorithms and moderation practices and provide detailed descriptions on how decisions are made, 2) commission independent audits of their algorithms, 3) solicit user feedback to identify potential biases or unintended consequences, 4) work collaboratively with researchers, civil society organizations, and stakeholders and provide more transparent data, and 5) publish regular reports on their practices.

Promoting digital literacy and critical thinking skills while providing more resources and support can help empower youth with intersectional identities to be mindful of their interactions and communications on social media and to make informed decisions about how they participate in the online world. Creating safe and equitable digital spaces for marginalized individuals to engage in self-representation, exploration, and connections is a crucial step toward improving youth mental health and well-being.

References

Abrams D, Hogg M: An Introduction to the Social Identity Approach. Birmingham, UK, Harvester-Wheatsheaf, 1990, pp 1–9

Abreu RL, Kenny MC: Cyberbullying and LGBTQ youth: a systematic literature review and recommendations for prevention and intervention. J Child Adolesc Trauma 11(1):81–97, 2017 32318140

Alhajji M, Bass S, Dai T: Cyberbullying, mental health, and violence in adolescents and associations with sex and race: data from the 2015 Youth Risk Behavior Survey. Glob Pediatr Health 6:2333794X19868887, 2019 31431904

Allen K-A, Ryan T, Gray D, et al: Social media use and social connectedness in adolescents: the positives and the potential pitfalls. Australian Journal of Educational and Developmental Psychology 31:18–31, 2014

Andalibi N, Lacombe-Duncan A, Roosevelt L, et al: LGBTQ persons' use of online spaces to navigate conception, pregnancy, and pregnancy loss: an intersectional approach. ACM Transactions on Computer-Human Interaction 29(1):1–46, 2022

Anti-Defamation League: Online Hate and Harassment: The American Experience. Washington, DC, Anti-Defamation League, February 11, 2019. Available at: https://www.adl.org/resources/report/online-hate-and-harassment-american-experience. Accessed January 24, 2023.

Arnett JJ, Žukauskienė R, Sugimura K: The new life stage of emerging adulthood at ages 18–29 years: implications for mental health. Lancet Psychiatry 1(7):569–576, 2014 26361316

Bell BT: Understanding adolescents, in Perspectives on HCI Research With Teenagers. Edited by Little L, Fitton D, Bell BT, et al. New York, Springer International, 2016, pp 11–27

Berger MN, Taba M, Marino JL, et al: Social media use and health and well-being of lesbian, gay, bisexual, transgender, and queer youth: systematic review. J Med Internet Res 24(9):e38449, 2022 36129741

Bivens R, Haimson OL: Baking gender into social media design: how platforms shape categories for users and advertisers. Soc Media Soc 2(4):2056305116672486, 2016

Black Lives Matter: 8 Years Strong. Black Lives Matter, July 13, 2021. Available at: https://blacklivesmatter.com/8-years-strong. Accessed February 27, 2023.

Bozzola E, Spina G, Agostiniani R, et al: The use of social media in children and adolescents: scoping review on the potential risks. Int J Environ Res Public Health 19(16):9960, 2022 36011593

Brown JJ: The hyperinvisibility of queer Black women in higher education. Master's thesis, Grand Valley State University, Allendale, MI, April 2021. Available at: https://scholarworks.gvsu.edu/cgi/viewcontent.cgi?article=2017&context=theses. Accessed December 4, 2023.

Brown M, Ray R, Summers E, et al: #SayHerName: a case study of intersectional social media activism. Ethn Racial Stud 40(11):1831–1846, 2017

Buckingham D (ed): Youth, Identity, and Digital Media. Cambridge, MA, MIT Press, 2007

Buolamwini J, Gebru T: Gender shades: intersectional accuracy disparities in commercial gender classification. Proceedings of the 1st Conference on Fairness, Accountability and Transparency 81:77–91, 2018

Cinelli M, De Francisci Morales G, Galeazzi A, et al: The echo chamber effect on social media. Proc Natl Acad Sci USA 118(9):e2023301118, 2021 33622786

Coleman B: Hello Avatar: Rise of the Networked Generation. Cambridge, MA, MIT Press, 2011

Collins PH, Bilge S: Intersectionality (Key Concepts). New York, Wiley, 2020

Cote AC: "I can defend myself": women's strategies for coping with harassment while gaming online. Games Cult 12(2):136–155, 2017

Crenshaw K: Demarginalizing the intersection of race and sex: a black feminist critique of antidiscrimination doctrine, feminist theory and antiracist politics. University of Chicago Legal Foundation 1(8):139–167, 1989

Crenshaw K: On Intersectionality: Essential Writings. New York, Faculty Books, 2017

de Vries KM: Intersectional identities and conceptions of the self: the experience of transgender people. Symbolic Interact 35(1):49–67, 2012

Eamon MK: Digital divide in computer access and use between poor and non-poor youth. J Soc Soc Welfare 31(2):91–112, 2004

Erikson EH: Identity: Youth and Crisis. New York, WW Norton, 1968

Evans JM: Exploring social media contexts for cultivating connected learning with Black youth in urban communities: the case of Dreamer Studio. Qual Sociol 45(3):393–411, 2022 35966136

Fosch-Villaronga E, Poulsen A, Søraa RA, et al: Gendering algorithms in social media. SIGKDD Explor 23(1):24–31, 2021

Francisco SC, Felmlee DH: What did you call me? An analysis of online harassment towards Black and Latinx women. Race Soc Probl 14(1):1–13, 2022

Gillespie T: Custodians of the Internet: Platforms, Content Moderation, and the Hidden Decisions That Shape Social Media. New Haven, CT, Yale University Press, 2018

GLAAD: Social Media Safety Index: 2022. New York, GLAAD, 2022. Available at: https://assets.glaad.org/m/29b001007886ae77/original/2022-GLAAD-Social-Media-Safety-Index.pdf. Accessed January 24, 2023.

Hawton K, Stewart A: Self-harm, suicidal behaviours, and cyberbullying in children and young people: systematic review. J Med Internet Res 20(4):1–15, 2018

Hinduja S, Patchin JW: Cyberbullying: an exploratory analysis of factors related to offending and victimization. Deviant Behav 29(2):129–156, 2008

Huang J, Kumar S, Hu C: A literature review of online identity reconstruction. Front Psychol 12:696552, 2021 34497560

Imana B, Korolova A, Heidemann J: Auditing for discrimination in algorithms delivering job ads. WWW '21: Proceedings of the Web Conference, Ljubljana, Slovenia, April 19–23, 2021, pp 3767–3778

Kaiser S, Kyrrestad H, Fossum S: Help-seeking behavior in Norwegian adolescents: the role of bullying and cyberbullying victimization in a cross-sectional study. Scand J Child Adolesc Psychiatry Psychol 8:81–90, 2020 33520780

Karizat N, Delmonaco D, Eslami M, et al: Algorithmic folk theories and identity: how TikTok users co-produce knowledge of identity and engage in algorithmic resistance. Proceedings of the ACM on Human-Computer Interaction 5(CSCW2):1–44, 2021

Keum BTH, Cano MÁ: Online racism, psychological distress, and alcohol use among racial minority women and men: a multi-group mediation analysis. Am J Orthopsychiatry 91(4):524–530, 2021 34338543

Litchfield C, Kavanagh E, Osborne J, et al: Social media and the politics of gender, race and identity: the case of Serena Williams. Eur J Sport Sci 15(2):154–170, 2018

Lorenz T: Internet "algospeak" is changing our language in real time, from "nip nops" to "le dollar bean." The Washington Post, April 8, 2022. Available at: https://www.washingtonpost.com/technology/2022/04/08/algospeak-tiktok-le-dollar-bean. Accessed December 4, 2023.

Matamoros-Fernández A, Farkas J: Racism, hate speech, and social media: a systematic review and critique. TV New Media 22(2):205–224, 2021

Mateu A, Pascual-Sánchez A, Martinez-Herves M, et al: Cyberbullying and post-traumatic stress symptoms in UK adolescents. Arch Dis Child 105(10):951–956, 2020 32576564

Maurya C, Muhammad T, Dhillon P, et al: The effects of cyberbullying victimization on depression and suicidal ideation among adolescents and young adults: a three year cohort study from India. BMC Psychiatry 22(1):599, 2022 36085004

McAdams DP: The Art and Science of Personality Development. New York, Guilford, 2015, pp xiv, 368

Metzler A, Scheithauer H: The long-term benefits of positive self-presentation via profile pictures, number of friends and the initiation of relationships on Facebook for adolescents' self-esteem and the initiation of offline relationships. Front Psychol 8:1981, 2017 29187827

National Academies of Sciences, Engineering, and Medicine, Division of Behavioral and Social Sciences and Education, Board on Children, Youth, and Families, et al: Adolescent Development, in The Promise of Adolescence: Realizing Opportunity for All Youth. Washington, DC, National Academies Press, 2019. Available at: https://www.ncbi.nlm.nih.gov/books/NBK545476. Accessed December 4, 2023.

Nelson R, Robards B, Churchill B, et al: Social media use among bisexuals and pansexuals: connection, harassment and mental health. Cult Health Sex 25(6):711–727, 2023 35900926

New Zealand Herald: #MyIdentity: prominent Kiwis involved in new social media campaign. New Zealand Herald, February 23, 2018. Available at: https://www.nzherald.co.nz/nz/myidentity-prominent-kiwis-involved-in-new-social-media-campaign/W7GVOXI4TU7QSJEA7QUOSH4QF4. Accessed February 28, 2023.

Noble SU: Algorithms of Oppression: How Search Engines Reinforce Racism. New York, NYU Press, 2018

Noble SU, Tynes BM (eds): The Intersectional Internet: Race, Sex, Class, and Culture Online. New York, Peter Lang, 2016

Obermaier M: Youth on standby? Explaining adolescent and young adult bystanders' intervention against online hate speech. New Media and Society 14614448221125416, 2022

Olayinka JT, Gohara MA, Ruffin QK: #BlackGirlMagic: impact of the social media movement on Black women's self esteem. Int J Womens Dermatol 7(2):171–173, 2021 33937485

Pasupathi M, Mansour E, Brubaker JR: Developing a life story: constructing relations between self and experience in autobiographical narratives. Hum Dev 50(2–3):85–110, 2007

Patchin JW, Hinduja S: Bullies move beyond the schoolyard: a preliminary look at cyberbullying. Youth Violence Juv Justice 4(2):148–169, 2006

Perloff RM: Social media effects on young women's body image concerns: theoretical perspectives and an agenda for research. Sex Roles 71(11):363–377, 2014

Qin Y, Lowe J: Is your online identity different from your offline identity? A study on the college students' online identities in China. Cult Psychol 27(1):67–95, 2021

Roberts ST: Behind the Screen: Content Moderation in the Shadows of Social Media. New Haven, CT, Yale University Press, 2019

Schemer C, Masur PK, Geiß S, et al: The impact of internet and social media use on well-being: a longitudinal analysis of adolescents across nine years. J Comput Mediat Commun 26(1):1–21, 2021

Selkie EM, Kota R, Chan Y-F, et al: Cyberbullying, depression, and problem alcohol use in female college students: a multisite study. Cyberpsychol Behav Soc Netw 18(2):79–86, 2015 25684608

Stieglitz S, Dang-Xuan L: Emotions and information diffusion in social media: sentiment of microblogs and sharing behavior. J Manage Inf Syst 29(4):217–247, 2013

Swart J: Experiencing algorithms: how young people understand, feel about, and engage with algorithmic news selection on social media. Social Media + Society 7(2):20563051211008828, 2021

Tynes BM, Mitchell KJ: Black youth beyond the digital divide: age and gender differences in internet use, communication patterns, and victimization experiences. J Black Psychol 40(3):291–307, 2014

Tynes BM, Giang MT, Williams DR, et al: Online racial discrimination and psychological adjustment among adolescents. J Adolesc Health 43(6):565–569, 2008 19027644

UNESCO: Addressing Hate Speech on Social Media: Contemporary Challenges. New York, United Nations Educational, Scientific, and Cultural Organization, 2021. Available at: https://unesdoc.unesco.org/ark:/48223/pf0000379177. Accessed February 14, 2023.

Uttarapong J, Cai J, Wohn DY: Harassment experiences of women and LGBTQ live streamers and how they handled negativity. Presented at IMX 2021—ACM International Conference on Interactive Media Experiences, 2021, pp 7–19

Vogels EA: Teens and cyberbullying 2022. Pew Research Center, December 15, 2022. Available at: https://www.pewresearch.org/internet/2022/12/15/teens-and-cyberbullying-2022. Accessed December 15, 2022.

World Advertising Research Center: Beyond Gender: The Impact of Intersectionality in Advertising. Available at: https://www.warc.com/content/paywall/article/warc-research/beyond-gender-the-impact-of-intersectionality-in-advertising/en-GB/149276. Accessed March 25, 2023.

Zhu C, Huang S, Evans R, et al: Cyberbullying among adolescents and children: a comprehensive review of the global situation, risk factors, and preventive measures. Front Public Health 9(March):634909, 2021 33791270

11

Body Image and Disordered Eating in Adolescence

Savannah R. Roberts, M.A.
Allegra R. Gordon, Sc.D., M.P.H.
Sophia Choukas-Bradley, Ph.D.

In this chapter, we address connections among social media use, body image concerns, and disordered eating, with an emphasis on adolescence—a developmental period characterized by high rates of social media use, body dissatisfaction, and disordered eating (Choukas-Bradley et al. 2022). We focus primarily on research with youth in Western nations, reflecting the current state of the literature. Given the global ubiquity of social media use, more research is needed in different cultural contexts.

Body image concerns and disordered eating are prevalent during adolescence. Population-based U.S. research suggests that approximately 57% of adolescent females and 31% of adolescent males engage in disordered eating (Simone et al. 2022), with 31% experiencing consistently high body dissatisfaction across adolescence (S.B. Wang et al. 2019). Social, biological, and cognitive transitions occur within a broader societal context that predisposes adolescents toward increased preoccupation with physical appearance and attractiveness. Meanwhile, the features of social media intersect with developmental processes and gendered sociocultural factors, creating a "perfect storm" for the emergence of body image concerns, particularly among adolescent females (Choukas-Bradley et al. 2022). Scholars have emphasized the need to move beyond a focus on screen time and toward a nuanced perspective on the specific social media experiences and identity factors that may confer risk (Hamilton et al. 2022).

Body Image Concerns and Disordered Eating During Adolescence

Adolescence is marked by substantial developmental changes that may increase risk for body dissatisfaction and disordered eating, especially among females. Peers are important for adolescents' sense of self, becoming the primary social reference group (Giletta et al. 2021). Adolescents experience a social-cognitive phenomenon called the "imaginary audience," believing peers are uniquely attuned to their behaviors and appearance (Elkind 1967; Giletta et al. 2021). In this context, a peer "appearance culture" often develops (Jones et al. 2004), and physical attractiveness often becomes a form of social capital (Mayeux and Kleiser 2020). Meanwhile, pubertal development leads to redistributions in fat, generally bringing female-bodied adolescents further from culturally established feminine beauty ideals that glamorize thinness, whereas male puberty increases musculature, aligning with masculine appearance ideals (Choukas-Bradley et al. 2022; Markey 2010). Less is known about the effects of puberty on gender minority adolescents' body image, but initial research indicates high levels of body dissatisfaction and disordered eating and the importance of access to gender-affirming care (e.g., Roberts et al. 2021; Romito et al. 2021).

Adolescent females are especially socialized to prioritize their physical appearance. According to the *tripartite influence model,* females are bombarded with messages from the media, parents, and peers regarding the importance of physical attractiveness (Thompson et al. 1999). According to *objectification theory* (Fredrickson and Roberts 1997), females learn to engage in self-objectification, internalizing an observer's perspective of their body. Adolescents may engage in disordered eating when they perceive a discrepancy between their body and the "ideal body" (Thompson et al. 1999). Furthermore, *weight stigma,* or negative stereotypes or evaluations of people in larger bodies, is a critical societal driver toward worse body image and disordered eating among all adolescents (Puhl and Latner 2007).

Given this reality, adolescents may mistakenly come to believe that they can achieve their ideal appearance by exerting control over their eating and exercise behaviors. These behaviors often align with sociocultural gendered appearance ideals, with young females most commonly engaging in disordered eating oriented toward femininity ideals (e.g., caloric restriction) and young males engaging in disordered eating oriented toward masculinity ideals (e.g., excess protein consumption, excessive weight lifting) (Murray 2017; Murray et al. 2016). It is critical to understand how transgender and gender-diverse adolescents may engage in disordered eating (Murray 2017) because initial research suggests that disordered eating may be motivated by a combination of gender identity concerns and weight and shape concerns (see Roberts et al. 2021; Romito et al. 2021).

> Sometimes I think about my feminine features, some of them on my face, some of them on my body. I mentioned before, like, my thighs. Some of them I can change through hormones and surgeries, but some of them I can't, really. I can't really change my hips. They may change a little bit if I am on hormones for a long time, but they will never really. I don't think my body will ever completely look like a cis man's body.
>
> *—trans male, nonbinary, age 16;*
> *they/them; assigned female at birth*

Research is sorely needed regarding how adolescents' racial and ethnic identities intersect with gender and sexual identities to affect body image. For example, culturally relevant appearance ideals such as hair and skin tone may be particularly relevant to the body image of youth of color, separately or in addition to the appearance dimensions of weight and shape (Ladd et al. 2022). Youth of color may navigate complex beauty ideals, shaped both by hegemonic Eurocentric standards of beauty and by identity-specific aspects of attractiveness (Ladd et al. 2022; Schooler 2008). Beauty ideals can be particularly challenging for young people with multiple marginalized social identities and positions, who must grapple with additional forms of prejudice, discrimination, and stigmatization in addition to weight stigma.

Social Media Use and Body Image Concerns in Adolescence

A review of four meta-analyses on experimental and longitudinal evidence regarding social media use and body image found some interesting results. When examined longitudinally, research generally only finds a small negative association between social media use (typically measured as frequency or duration of use) and body image (de Valle et al. 2021). However, experimental research, which typically manipulates the type of content participants view, repeatedly demonstrates a robust negative effect of viewing appearance-focused content (e.g., edited photos or videos of peers and celebrities on platforms such as Instagram or TikTok) on participants' body image (de Valle et al. 2021). In line with these results, emerging evidence underscores the importance of examining adolescents' specific social media experiences rather than their overall time spent on social media (Choukas-Bradley et al. 2022; Hamilton et al. 2022). We proposed a developmental-sociocultural theoretical framework for how specific social media features and experiences may exacerbate adolescent females' body image concerns and, in turn, their disordered eating (Choukas-Bradley et al. 2022). In this model, we addressed how social media experiences may intersect with developmental and gendered sociocultural processes to create a "perfect storm" for body image concerns among some females (Choukas-Bradley et al. 2022). Specifically, we argued that social media use may increase young females' problematic focus on both other people's and their own physical appearance (Choukas-Bradley et al. 2022). For example, in related empirical work, we found that adolescent females feel appearance pressure from using social media, pressure associated with internalization of thin and muscular beauty ideals (Roberts et al. 2022). We also addressed the construct of *appearance-related social media consciousness* (ASMC), which reflects preoccupation with one's appearance to a social media audience (Choukas-Bradley et al. 2019, 2020). Furthermore, we proposed that the "imaginary audience" may no longer be imaginary in this era (Choukas-Bradley et al. 2022). In the discussion that follows, we describe specific social media experiences that have shown consistent associations with body image concerns.

Selfies

Adolescents commonly take, edit, and post photos of themselves (McLean et al. 2019). Economists believe that the proliferation of selfies on social media is likely related to the mass-marketing of smartphones with front-facing cameras and the growth of image-based platforms such as Instagram (Senft and Baym 2015). Importantly, the "selfie phenomenon" has had a noticeable impact on brands' marketing strategies, which use them as advertisements to display their product in a subtle manner that suggests authenticity and trustworthiness (Lim 2016). As such, adolescents on social media are embedded in a capitalistic system in which brands are invested in increasing selfie activity for their marketing purposes and profit margins.

However, these behaviors may encourage youth to view their appearance from an observer's perspective, imagining how they will be judged by a public audience (Choukas-Bradley et al. 2020, 2022). Among teens, ASMC—or worrying about how one appears to their audience—is associated with body surveillance, body shame, body comparison, and disordered eating (Choukas-Bradley et al. 2020). The cognitive experience of ASMC could be an underlying reason that taking and editing selfies is associated with adolescents' self-objectification in the United States (Meier and Gray 2014) and China (Zheng et al. 2019). Furthermore, appearance comparison may be a mechanism linking selfie activities to body image concerns (Mingoia et al. 2019). Lastly, people who frequently post selfies have higher levels of body dissatisfaction, shape and weight concerns, internalization of the thin ideal, body shame, and restrained eating relative to peers who post them less often or never (McLean et al. 2015; Salomon and Brown 2019; Wilksch et al. 2020).

Photo Editing

Photo editing is common among adolescents, particularly females (McLean et al. 2015), who spend hours meticulously editing their images (Chua and Chang 2016; Yau and Reich 2019). In 2015, the photo-editing application (app) Facetune reported $18 million in revenue; in 2017, it became Apple's most popular paid app (Bort 2015; Jennings 2019; Solon 2018). During the early days of the coronavirus disease 2019 (COVID-19) pandemic, the time people spent on photo-editing apps increased by 20%, and the user base of these apps tripled (Brown 2020).

The ability to edit one's appearance in photos is particularly problematic for adolescents' body image and their risk for developing disordered eating. Photo editing encourages adolescents to scrutinize their appearance for perceived flaws, then "fix" them by applying filters and photo manipulations. Adolescents may not recognize the alteration in others' edited photos, falsely believing that they are "realistic," while simultaneously preferring them to unedited photos (Kleemans et al. 2018). Photo editing is associated with adolescents' self-objectification and subsequent appearance anxiety, body shame (Terán et al. 2020), and body image concerns (Y. Wang et al. 2019). Furthermore, disclaimers on edited photos are ineffective in protecting body satisfaction (Tiggemann 2022).

Likes and Comments

Adolescents often post images in hopes of receiving likes and comments—numeric indicators of peer status (Nesi et al. 2018). As such, likes and comments become a form of appearance-related feedback that likely influences their body image (Choukas-Bradley et al. 2022). Providing this feedback or liking and commenting on others' content is associated with decreased appearance of self-esteem across adolescence (Steinsbekk et al. 2021). Viewing likes and comments on others' photos is associated with social comparison (Fardouly et al. 2017; Fox and Vendemia 2016). Among adolescents, receiving comments on social media about one's appearance is associated with self-objectification (Slater and Tiggemann 2015), qualitative descriptions of depressive feelings, and lower self-esteem (Berne et al. 2014).

Influencers

Influencers are individuals who have amassed a large social media following and often profit financially from brand partnerships and sponsored posts. These individuals are often young and conventionally attractive and are thought of as regular or relatable peers. As such, adolescents may compare themselves with influencers, whose appearance may seem attainable (Choukas-Bradley et al. 2022). Influencers are then easily able to market products and services to teens in a manner that seems authentic and genuine (Vrontis et al. 2021), like a friend making a recommendation. Because influencers are paid by the number of likes, comments, and shares their posts receive (Vrontis et al. 2021), they are incentivized to garner as much attention as possible. Adolescents report personally relating to influencers, whose content (including sponsored advertisements) is routinely integrated into their everyday lives (de Castro et al. 2021). To date, little research has been done examining the specific effects of influencers on adolescents' body image and risk for disordered eating. However, influencers represent an important area for future research in the body image and disordered eating fields.

Harmful Body- and Eating-Related Social Media Content

Thinspiration and *fitspiration* are terms used to describe images on social media that display either ultrathin individuals with messaging that promotes weight loss (Ghaznavi and Taylor 2015) or thin and toned individuals who promote exercise and dieting (Tiggemann and Zaccardo 2018). Even brief exposure to this content is associated with worse body image among young adult females (Prnjak et al. 2020; Rounds and Stutts 2021), and effects are likely similar among adolescents. These messages promote disordered eating by encouraging caloric restriction and excessive exercise to achieve unattainable appearance ideals (Harris et al. 2018). Body ideals are culturally constructed and change over time, and exposure to any type of idealized and unrealistic beauty standard may promote body dissatisfaction and increase vulnerability to eating disorders. For example, an experimental study found that exposure to "slim-thick" imagery (featuring a small waist but large hips, buttocks, and thighs) was even more strongly predictive of young women's body dissatisfaction than was exposure to thin-ideal imagery (McComb and Mills 2022).

In one notable trend, individuals share #WhatIEatInADay videos on TikTok and YouTube, posting their daily food intake. Little research has examined this trend's effects on body image and disordered eating. However, a preliminary investigation showed that much of the content glorifies weight loss and lacks credible nutrition information (Minadeo and Pope 2022). Adolescents also are bombarded by food-, body-, and beauty-related advertisements on social media; many companies use it to sell weight-loss and muscle-building supplements, which poses a danger to adolescent health (Pomeranz et al. 2015). Individuals who engage in disordered eating are more likely to search for content about weight loss and fitness (Carrotte et al. 2015). The terms "pro-ana" and "pro-mia" (for "pro-anorexia" and "pro-bulimia," respectively) refer to content specifically designed to encourage eating disorders, including images that inspire extreme thinness, techniques for caloric restriction, and messages promoting anti-recovery (Bert et al. 2016). Pro–eating disorder profiles are primarily followed by adolescent females (Bert et al. 2016) and may be related to the etiology of eating disorders, particularly among this population (Mento et al. 2021). One report found that when adolescent females search for weight loss or dieting information, algorithms may lead them toward these pro–disordered eating sites (Tech Transparency Project 2021).

Potential for Social Media to Improve Body Image

Some emerging research focuses on social media's potential for improving body image and reducing vulnerability to disordered eating. The "body positive" movement purportedly aims to improve body image by depicting a broader range of sizes and appearances as attractive, compared with the typical "thin ideal" media. However, a review of experimental studies found that exposure to body-positive media has mixed effects (Fioravanti et al. 2022). Body-positive content may be beneficial for individuals' body image if they explicitly seek it out themselves (Kvardova et al. 2022), curating their own feeds to include more attainable appearance ideals. It is also possible that seeking out body-positive content is simply a marker of positive body image. However, body-positive media often portrays larger females in a sexualized manner, thereby contributing to sexual objectification (Cohen et al. 2019). Experimental work also suggests that brief exposure to body-positive content may increase *both* body satisfaction and self-objectification (Cohen et al. 2019).

It is important to note that body-positive media still maintains an appearance focus, perhaps reinforcing the notion that a person's worth is determined by their attractiveness. Alternative movements have arisen, such as *body neutrality* (which maintains an appearance-neutral focus) and *body functionality* (which focuses on what the body allows an individual to accomplish, rather than its appearance). A scoping review of body-positive social media content concluded that non-appearance-focused posts, such as text-based posts promoting body acceptance or images of plants, animals, travel, and landscapes, may be most beneficial for promoting positive body image (Rodgers et al. 2021).

Practice and Policy Implications

Ecological systems theory has received robust empirical support for decades emphasizing the importance of considering the multitude of settings that impact child and adolescent development (Bronfenbrenner 1977). To reduce adolescents' vulnerability to body dissatisfaction and eating disorders associated with their social media use, interventions that target multiple settings are likely to be most effective. Because social media affects almost the entire youth population, individual-level interventions may be less fruitful than societal ones. Public health approaches to combat disordered eating are sorely needed (Austin 2012). In the following section, and in Figure 11–1, we summarize clinical and policy recommendations for adolescent use of social media.

Clinical Recommendations

Adults who interact directly with youth (e.g., their parents, family members, guardians, clinicians, teachers, coaches, religious leaders) can be influential and should consider ways to leverage the youth's social media use to reduce their risk for eating disorders and improve their body image. We recommend that clinicians and caretakers focus on *how* adolescents are using social media, rather than on their overall screen time. If an adolescent is struggling with body dissatisfaction or disordered eating, clinicians should assess whether the adolescent is engaging with features that may promote

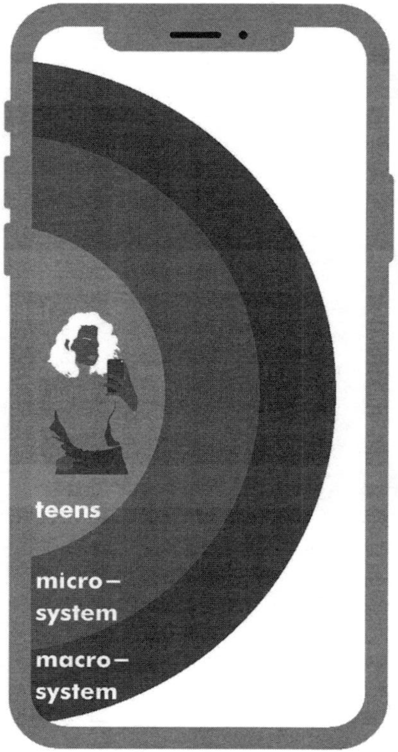

Practice and Policy Recommendations

Teens

- Encourage teens to monitor how their social media use makes them feel and to curate their content to show material that enhances their self-esteem and feelings of social connection
- Discourage teens from seeking out dieting and exercise-related content
- Embolden teens to develop social media literacy

Microsystem

- Clinicians ought to assess whether teens are engaging with social media features known to be associated with body image concerns, such as photo-editing and exposure to fitspiration and thinspiration
- Parents ought to discuss marketing tactics with adolescents to prevent purchasing of weight- and muscle-building supplements and products
- Educators should consider offering classroom-based social media literacy interventions

Macrosystem (Policies, Social Media Environment)

- Implement public health approaches to eating disorder prevention
- Increase investment in research on social media and youth mental health
- Develop regulations for protecting adolescents from social media features associated with body image concerns and disordered eating
- Fund programs that support critical media literacy in school settings, with a focus on digital literacy
- Require social media companies to be more transparent with researchers, policymakers, and advocates invested in youth mental health
- Develop state and federal safety standards for online services

teens

micro—
system

macro—
system

Figure 11–1. Practice and policy recommendations for adolescents' social media use.

body image concerns (e.g., photo editing, exposure to idealized bodies). Adolescents should then be encouraged to curate their profiles/feeds in a way that promotes positive body image. In addition, some research finds that parental support and positive school climates can shape adolescent females' interactions with social media (Burnette et al. 2017). In environments that implicitly and explicitly encourage self-acceptance and valuing diversity, they describe being better able to contend with appearance-related content (Burnette et al. 2017).

Adults can also promote social media literacy, which enhances adolescents' abilities to think critically about it. Social media literacy interventions have shown promise in the classroom (McLean et al. 2017), and a cluster randomized controlled trial is underway to determine their effectiveness (Gordon et al. 2020). Importantly, it may be protective for young females' body image (Paxton et al. 2022), but more research is needed to understand how we can best serve the needs of young males and gender-diverse youth. It is possible that platforms could offer support to youth struggling with body image or eating disorders, although more research is needed. A randomized controlled trial found that a chatbot (i.e., a computer program that simulates human conversation) based on an evidenced-based cognitive-behavioral eating disorders prevention program was successful in reducing adult females' concerns about weight and shape, their overall eating disorder pathology, and their likelihood of eating disorder onset (Fitzsimmons-Craft et al. 2022). This promising intervention should be tested in adolescents. With regard to eating disorder recovery communities on social media, initial evidence suggests they may contain unhelpful content and are sometimes used in place of professional treatment (Au and Cosh 2022). However, because social media is already being used by most adolescents and offers a highly accessible, cost-effective medium for finding support, future work should assess how platforms can best promote positive body image and prevent disordered eating.

Policy Recommendations

Given the influence of the technology and beauty industries that engineer and profit from social media, we need policies that address its potential deleterious effects on youth body image and disordered eating, as well as policies that promote potential benefits of its use. Unfortunately, little research has been done on these potential policy approaches. One small qualitative study in the United Kingdom found that parents were interested in schools playing a key role as providers of digital education and prevention, emphasizing a desire for media literacy programming that goes beyond online safety (Throuvala et al. 2021).

Research on cost-effectiveness of macro-level preventive interventions for eating disorders also offers relevant insights. One study using advanced simulation modeling techniques found that universal prevention interventions to reduce the societal burden of eating disorders are likely to be cost-saving from a public health perspective (Long et al. 2022). Particular cost savings were identified for 1) a school-based universal preventive intervention that included media use behaviors and 2) legal restriction banning sale of over-the-counter diet pills to youth (Long et al. 2022).

Policy efforts thus far have had mixed results. In 2019, Facebook/Instagram (now Meta) initiated a "voluntary" ban of weight-loss products following widespread backlash from youth advocates and celebrities (Rosenbloom 2019). However, targeting youth with harmful advertising content continued (e.g., extreme dieting ads) (Tech Transparency Project 2021). Even after Meta announced it would end the targeting of advertising to minors (Culliford 2021), further investigation uncovered new youth-targeted advertising (Ho and Farthing 2021). These findings underscore the need to implement more effective regulatory and policy approaches for reducing potentially harmful content.

Several potential policy approaches have been proposed by professional societies, scholars, advocacy groups, federal agencies, and policymakers with the goal of addressing links between youth social media use and body image. For example, the 2021 U.S. Surgeon General's Advisory *Protecting Youth Mental Health* called for all levels of government to be involved in protecting youth mental health in online environments, including social media. In the following list we highlight several policy approaches that have been suggested to spur macro-level changes that could directly or indirectly disrupt links between youth social media use and disordered eating:

- *Increase investment in research on social media and youth mental health.* For several years calls have been made for a stronger research agenda on social media and public health (Pagoto et al. 2019; U.S. Surgeon General 2021). This agenda must advance research on macro-level interventions, including policy implementation and barriers, cost-effectiveness, and youth perspectives. Policy initiatives needing evaluation include protections against manipulative advertising and marketing content (Federal Trade Commission 2022), including monitoring the use of influencers for advertising products to minors (LaCasse 2022). The Center of Excellence is one such example of a federally funded center for advancing research and policy in these areas (American Academy of Pediatrics 2023).

- *Fund programs that support critical media literacy instruction in school settings, with a particular focus on the unique properties of digital media.* Media literacy advocates argue for and track the progress of state-level media literacy policies (Bulger and Davison 2018). Free, age-specific curricula exist for teaching students broadly about digital media (Common Sense Education 2023). However, research is needed to define key outcomes and to evaluate which forms of media literacy education are (or are not) effective in promoting positive body image development or reducing disordered eating behaviors, specifically.

- *Require companies to be more transparent.* Scholars have argued for the importance of increasing transparency regarding the "black box" algorithms that determine what content is offered to youth users, including giving users more control over how their personal data and other "inputs" are used (Giansiracusa 2021). The Surgeon General's Advisory goes further by recommending policies that would require social media platforms to disclose meaningful data for research purposes and enable systematic auditing of platform algorithms (U.S. Surgeon General 2021). Furthermore, policymakers are now considering various strategies for reducing harm from algorithms (Holdheim 2022).

- *Develop state and federal safety standards for online services.* It is crucial that platforms be designed with developmental considerations in mind. New safety standards might include, for example, standards or restrictions regarding data collection, age verification, engagement techniques (e.g., "nudges," extreme content), and youth-targeted advertising (U.S. Surgeon General 2021). Notable examples include the United Kingdom's Age-Appropriate Design Code (U.K. Information Commissioner's Office 2022), the Australian government's Safety by Design initiatives (eSafety Commissioner 2022), and the California Age-Appropriate Design Code Bill (5Rights Foundation 2022). The U.K. initiative has led to product changes to better protect users' rights, safety, and privacy by companies such as Instagram, TikTok, and YouTube (Lomas 2021).

Conclusion

Researchers have identified a number of appearance-focused features on social media that are associated with body image concerns and disordered eating. Given the prevalence of body dissatisfaction and eating pathology during adolescence, it is critical that researchers and policymakers collaborate to protect youth mental and physical health. Research remains limited on clinical and policy interventions to disrupt harmful pathways between social media experiences and eating disorders. Despite this scarcity, advocates for youth mental health have advanced several clinical and policy approaches for reducing adolescents' vulnerability to body image concerns and eating pathology. Future research must evaluate emerging social media interventions to determine their effectiveness in alleviating the burden of body dissatisfaction and disordered eating among all youth, while taking into account adolescents' intersecting racial, ethnic, sex/gender, and sexual identities and related systems of social inequality, as well as the technology and appearance industries' drive for profit over adolescent health and well-being.

References

American Academy of Pediatrics: Center of Excellence on Social Media and Youth Mental Health. Washington, DC, American Academy of Pediatrics, September 15, 2023. Available at: https://www.aap.org/en/patient-care/media-and-children/center-of-excellence-on-social-media-and-youth-mental-health. Accessed April 30, 2024.

Au ES, Cosh SM: Social media and eating disorder recovery: an exploration of Instagram recovery community users and their reasons for engagement. Eat Behav 46(August):101651, 2022 35760017

Austin SB: A public health approach to eating disorders prevention: it's time for public health professionals to take a seat at the table. BMC Public Health 12(1):854, 2012 23043459

Berne S, Frisén A, Kling J: Appearance-related cyberbullying: a qualitative investigation of characteristics, content, reasons, and effects. Body Image 11(4):527–533, 2014 25194309

Bert F, Gualano MR, Camussi E, et al: Risks and threats of social media websites: Twitter and the proana movement. Cyberpsychol Behav Soc Netw 19(4):233–238, 2016 26991868

Bort J: How the makers of Facetune raked in ~$18 million in 2 years and caught Facebook's eye. Business Insider, August 18, 2015. Available at: https://www.businessinsider.com/how-the-makers-of-facetune-raked-at-least-18-million-in-under-two-years-and-caught-facebooks-eye-2015-8. Accessed December 4, 2023.

Bronfenbrenner U: Toward an experimental ecology of human development. Am Psychol 32(7):513–531, 1977

Brown D: "Your roots are showing": photo editing apps surge after salons shut down amid coronavirus. USA Today, April 1, 2020. Available at: https://www.usatoday.com/story/tech/2020/04/01/coronavirus-photo-video-editing-apps-surge/5087790002. Accessed December 4, 2023.

Bulger M, Davison P: The promises, challenges, and futures of media literacy. J Media Lit Educ 10(1):1–21, 2018

Burnette CB, Kwitowski MA, Mazzeo SE: "I don't need people to tell me I'm pretty on social media": a qualitative study of social media and body image in early adolescent girls. Body Image 23(December):114–125, 2017 28965052

Carrotte ER, Vella AM, Lim MS: Predictors of "liking" three types of health and fitness-related content on social media: a cross-sectional study. J Med Internet Res 17(8):e205, 2015 26297689

Choukas-Bradley S, Nesi J, Widman L, et al: Camera-ready: young women's appearance-related social media consciousness. Psychol Pop Media Cult 8(4):473–481, 2019

Choukas-Bradley S, Nesi J, Widman L, et al: The Appearance-Related Social Media Consciousness Scale: development and validation with adolescents. Body Image 33(June):164–174, 2020 32193170

Choukas-Bradley S, Roberts SR, Maheux AJ, et al: The perfect storm: a developmental-sociocultural framework for the role of social media in adolescent girls' body image concerns and mental health. Clin Child Fam Psychol Rev 25(4):681–701, 2022 35841501

Chua THH, Chang L: Follow me and like my beautiful selfies: Singapore teenage girls' engagement in self-presentation and peer comparison on social media. Comput Human Behav 55(February):190–197, 2016

Cohen R, Fardouly J, Newton-John T, et al: #BoPo on Instagram: an experimental investigation of the effects of viewing body positive content on young women's mood and body image. New Media Soc 21(7):1546–1564, 2019

Common Sense Education: Everything You Need to Teach Digital Citizenship. San Francisco, CA, Common Sense Education, 2023. Available at: https://www.commonsense.org/education/digital-citizenship. Accessed January 25, 2023.

Culliford E: Facebook will restrict ad targeting of under-18s. Reuters, July 27, 2021. Available at: https://www.reuters.com/technology/facebook-will-restrict-ad-targeting-under-18s-2021-07-27. Accessed December 4, 2023.

de Castro CA, O'Reilly I, Carthy A: Social media influencers (SMIs) in context: a literature review. Journal of Marketing Management 9(2):59–71, 2021

de Valle MK, Gallego-García M, Williamson P, et al: Social media, body image, and the question of causation: meta-analyses of experimental and longitudinal evidence. Body Image 39(December):276–292, 2021 34695681

Elkind D: Egocentrism in adolescence. Child Dev 38(4):1025–1034, 1967 5583052

eSafety Commissioner: Safety by design. Sydney, Australian Government, 2022. https://www.esafety.gov.au/industry/safety-by-design. Accessed January 25, 2023.

Fardouly J, Pinkus RT, Vartanian LR: The impact of appearance comparisons made through social media, traditional media, and in person in women's everyday lives. Body Image 20(March):31–39, 2017 27907812

Federal Trade Commission: Protecting Kids From Stealth Advertising in Digital Media. Washington, DC, Federal Trade Commission, 2022. Available at: https://www.ftc.gov/news-events/events/2022/10/protecting-kids-stealth-advertising-digital-media. Accessed January 25, 2023.

Fioravanti G, Benucci SB, Ceragioli G, et al: How the exposure to beauty ideals on social networking sites influences body image: a systematic review of experimental studies. Adolesc Res Rev 7(7):419–458, 2022

Fitzsimmons-Craft EE, Chan WW, Smith AC, et al: Effectiveness of a chatbot for eating disorders prevention: a randomized clinical trial. Int J Eat Disord 55(3):343–353, 2022 35274362

5Rights Foundation: California Age Appropriate Design Code. March 18, 2022. Available at: https://5rightsfoundation.com/uploads/California-Age-Appropriate-Design-Code_short-briefing.pdf. Accessed December 4, 2023.

Fox J, Vendemia MA: Selective self-presentation and social comparison through photographs on social networking sites. Cyberpsychol Behav Soc Netw 19(10):593–600, 2016 27732079

Fredrickson BL, Roberts T-A: Objectification theory. Psychol Women Q 21(2):173–206, 1997

Ghaznavi J, Taylor LD: Bones, body parts, and sex appeal: an analysis of #thinspiration images on popular social media. Body Image 14(June):54–61, 2015 25880783

Giansiracusa N: How Algorithms Create and Prevent Fake News: Exploring the Impacts of Social Media, Deepfakes, GPT-3, and More. Berkeley, CA, Apress, 2021

Giletta M, Choukas-Bradley S, Maes M, et al: A meta-analysis of longitudinal peer influence effects in childhood and adolescence. Psychol Bull 147(7):719–747, 2021 34855429

Gordon CS, Rodgers RF, Slater AE, et al: A cluster randomized controlled trial of the SoMe social media literacy body image and wellbeing program for adolescent boys and girls: study protocol. Body Image 33(June):27–37, 2020 32086189

Hamilton JL, Nesi J, Choukas-Bradley S: Reexamining social media and socioemotional well-being among adolescents through the lens of the COVID-19 pandemic: a theoretical review and directions for future research. Perspect Psychol Sci 17(3):662–679, 2022 34756118

Harris JK, Duncan A, Men V, et al: Messengers and messages for tweets that used #thinspo and #fitspo hashtags in 2016. Prev Chronic Dis 15(January):E01, 2018 29300696

Ho EY-C, Farthing R: How Facebook Still Targets Surveillance Ads to Teens. Sydney, Reset Australia, November 2021. Available at: https://fairplayforkids.org/wp-content/uploads/2021/11/fbsurveillancereport.pdf. Accessed December 4, 2023.

Holdheim S: Regulating Content Recommendation Algorithms in Social Media. Yale University Thurman Arnold Project, May 11, 2022. Available at: https://som.yale.edu/sites/default/files/2022-05/DPRC-Holdheim.pdf. Accessed December 4, 2023.

Jennings R: Facetune and the internet's endless pursuit of physical perfection. Vox, July 16, 2019. Available at: https://www.vox.com/the-highlight/2019/7/16/20689832/instagram-photo-editing-app-facetune. Accessed December 4, 2023.

Jones DC, Vigfusdottir TH, Lee Y: Body image and the appearance culture among adolescent girls and boys: an examination of friend conversations, peer criticism, appearance magazines, and the internalization of appearance ideals. J Adolesc Res 19(3):323–339, 2004

Kleemans M, Daalmans S, Carbaat I, et al: Picture perfect: the direct effect of manipulated Instagram photos on body image in adolescent girls. Media Psychol 21(1):93–110, 2018

Kvardova N, Machackova H, Smahel D: A moderated mediation model for body-positive online content and body image among adolescents. Body Image 42(September):370–374, 2022 35930872

LaCasse A: FTC Event on Digital Advertising to Children Looks at Brand-Influencer Relationships. Portsmouth, NH, The International Association of Privacy Professionals, 2022. Available at: https://iapp.org/news/a/ftc-panels-on-digital-advertising-to-children-focuses-on-disclosures-of-brand-influencer-relationships. Accessed December 4, 2023.

Ladd BA, Maheux AJ, Roberts SR, et al: Black adolescents' appearance concerns, depressive symptoms, and self-objectification: exploring the roles of gender and ethnic-racial identity commitment. Body Image 43(December):314–325, 2022 36242995

Lim WM: Understanding the selfie phenomenon: current insights and future research directions. Eur J Mark 50(9/10):1773–1788, 2016

Lomas N: UK now expects compliance with Children's Privacy Design Code. TechCrunch, September 1, 2021. Available at: https://techcrunch.com/2021/09/01/uk-now-expects-compliance-with-its-child-privacy-design-code. Accessed December 4, 2023.

Long MW, Ward ZJ, Wright DR, et al: Cost-effectiveness of 5 public health approaches to prevent eating disorders. Am J Prev Med 63(6):935–943, 2022 36109308

Markey CN: Invited commentary: why body image is important to adolescent development. J Youth Adolesc 39(12):1387–1391, 2010 20339908

Mayeux L, Kleiser M: A gender prototypicality theory of adolescent peer popularity. Adolesc Res Rev 5(3):295–306, 2020

McComb SE, Mills JS: Eating and body image characteristics of those who aspire to the slim-thick, thin, or fit ideal and their impact on state body image. Body Image 42(September):375–384, 2022 35930873

McLean SA, Paxton SJ, Wertheim EH, et al: Photoshopping the selfie: self photo editing and photo investment are associated with body dissatisfaction in adolescent girls. Int J Eat Disord 48(8):1132–1140, 2015 26311205

McLean SA, Wertheim EH, Masters J, et al: A pilot evaluation of a social media literacy intervention to reduce risk factors for eating disorders. Int J Eat Disord 50(7):847–851, 2017 28370321

McLean SA, Jarman HK, Rodgers RF: How do "selfies" impact adolescents' well-being and body confidence? A narrative review. Psychol Res Behav Manag 12(July):513–521, 2019 31372071

Meier EP, Gray J: Facebook photo activity associated with body image disturbance in adolescent girls. Cyberpsychol Behav Soc Netw 17(4):199–206, 2014 24237288

Mento C, Silvestri MC, Muscatello MRA, et al: Psychological impact of pro-anorexia and pro-eating disorder websites on adolescent females: a systematic review. Int J Environ Res Public Health 18(4):2186, 2021 33672305

Minadeo M, Pope L: Weight-normative messaging predominates on TikTok: a qualitative content analysis. PLoS One 17(11):e0267997, 2022 36318532

Mingoia J, Hutchinson AD, Gleaves DH, et al: The impact of a social media literacy intervention on positive attitudes to tanning: a pilot study. Comput Human Behav 90(January):188–195, 2019

Murray SB: Gender identity and eating disorders: the need to delineate novel pathways for eating disorder symptomatology. J Adolesc Health 60(1):1–2, 2017 27838236

Murray SB, Griffiths S, Mond JM: Evolving eating disorder psychopathology: conceptualising muscularity-oriented disordered eating. Br J Psychiatry 208(5):414–415, 2016 27143005

Nesi J, Choukas-Bradley S, Prinstein MJ: Transformation of adolescent peer relations in the social media context, part 1: a theoretical framework and application to dyadic peer relationships. Clin Child Fam Psychol Rev 21(3):267–294, 2018 29627907

Pagoto S, Waring ME, Xu R: A call for a public health agenda for social media research. J Med Internet Res 21(12):e16661, 2019 31855185

Paxton SJ, McLean SA, Rodgers RF: "My critical filter buffers your app filter": social media literacy as a protective factor for body image. Body Image 40(March):158–164, 2022 34968853

Pomeranz JL, Barbosa G, Killian C, et al: The dangerous mix of adolescents and dietary supplements for weight loss and muscle building: legal strategies for state action. J Public Health Manag Pract 21(5):496–503, 2015 25248073

Prnjak K, Pemberton S, Helms E, et al: Reactions to ideal body shapes. J Gen Psychol 147(4):361–380, 2020 31608821

Puhl RM, Latner JD: Stigma, obesity, and the health of the nation's children. Psychol Bull 133(4):557–580, 2007 17592956

Roberts SR, Salk RH, Thoma BC, et al: Disparities in disordered eating between gender minority and cisgender adolescents. Int J Eat Disord 54(7):1135–1146, 2021 33638569

Roberts SR, Maheux AJ, Hunt RA, et al: Incorporating social media and muscular ideal internalization into the tripartite influence model of body image: towards a modern understanding of adolescent girls' body dissatisfaction. Body Image 41(June):239–247, 2022 35306356

Rodgers RF, Paxton SJ, Wertheim EH: #Take idealized bodies out of the picture: a scoping review of social media content aiming to protect and promote positive body image. Body Image 38(September):10–36, 2021 33798800

Romito M, Salk RH, Roberts SR, et al: Exploring transgender adolescents' body image concerns and disordered eating: semi-structured interviews with nine gender minority youth. Body Image 37(June):50–62, 2021 33549975

Rosenbloom C: Instagram and Facebook ban "miracle" diet posts, but there's much more work to do. The Washington Post, September 24, 2019. Available at: https://www.washingtonpost.com/lifestyle/wellness/instagram-and-facebook-ban-miracle-diet-posts-but-theres-much-more-work-to-do/2019/09/23/0829a872-de26-11e9-b199-f638bf2c340f_story.html. Accessed December 4, 2023.

Rounds EG, Stutts LA: The impact of fitspiration content on body satisfaction and negative mood: an experimental study. Psychology of Popular Media 10:267–274, 2021

Salomon I, Brown CS: The selfie generation: examining the relationship between social media use and early adolescent body image. J Early Adolesc 39(4):539–560, 2019

Schooler D: Real women have curves: a longitudinal investigation of TV and the body image development of Latina adolescents. J Adolesc Res 23(2):132–153, 2008

Senft TM, Baym NK: What does the selfie say? Investigating a global phenomenon. International Journal of Communication 9:1588–1606, 2015

Simone M, Telke S, Anderson LM, et al: Ethnic/racial and gender differences in disordered eating behavior prevalence trajectories among women and men from adolescence into adulthood. Soc Sci Med 294(February):114720, 2022 35033795

Slater A, Tiggemann M: Media exposure, extracurricular activities, and appearance-related comments as predictors of female adolescents' self-objectification. Psychol Women Q 39(3):375–389, 2015

Solon O: FaceTune is conquering Instagram: but does it take airbrushing too far? The Guardian, March 9, 2018. Available at: https://www.theguardian.com/media/2018/mar/09/facetune-photoshopping-app-instagram-body-image-debate. Accessed December 4, 2023.

Steinsbekk S, Wichstrøm L, Stenseng F, et al: The impact of social media use on appearance self-esteem from childhood to adolescence: a 3-wave community study. Comput Human Behav 114(January):106528, 2021

Tech Transparency Project: "Thinstagram": Instagram's algorithm fuels eating disorder epidemic. Tech Transparency Project, December 8, 2021. Available at: https://www.techtransparencyproject.org/articles/thinstagram-instagrams-algorithm-fuels-eating-disorder-epidemic. Accessed December 4, 2023.

Terán L, Yan K, Aubrey JS: "But first let me take a selfie": U.S. adolescent girls' selfie activities, self-objectification, imaginary audience beliefs, and appearance concerns. J Child Media 14(3):343–360, 2020

Thompson JK, Heinberg LJ, Altabe M, et al: Exacting Beauty: Theory, Assessment, and Treatment of Body Image Disturbance. Washington, DC, American Psychological Association, 1999

Throuvala MA, Griffiths MD, Rennoldson M, et al: Policy recommendations for preventing problematic internet use in schools: a qualitative study of parental perspectives. Int J Environ Res Public Health 18(9):4522, 2021 33923208

Tiggemann M: Digital modification and body image on social media: disclaimer labels, captions, hashtags, and comments. Body Image 41(June):172–180, 2022 35259655

Tiggemann M, Zaccardo M: "Strong is the new skinny": a content analysis of #fitspiration images on Instagram. J Health Psychol 23(8):1003–1011, 2018 27611630

U.K. Information Commissioner's Office: Introduction to the Age Appropriate Design Code. London, UK Information Commissioner's Office, 2022. Available at: https://ico.org.uk/for-organisations/guide-to-data-protection/ico-codes-of-practice/age-appropriate-design-code. Accessed January 25, 2023.

U.S. Surgeon General: Protecting Youth Mental Health: The U.S. Surgeon General's Advisory. Washington DC, U.S. Department of Health and Human Services, 2021. Available at: https://www.hhs.gov/sites/default/files/surgeon-general-youth-mental-health-advisory.pdf. Accessed January 25, 2023.

Vrontis D, Makrides A, Christofi M, et al: Social media influencer marketing: a systematic review, integrative framework, and future research agenda. Int J Consum Stud 45(4):617–644, 2021

Wang SB, Haynos AF, Wall MM, et al: Fifteen-year prevalence, trajectories, and predictors of body dissatisfaction from adolescence to middle adulthood. Clin Psychol Sci 7(6):1403–1415, 2019 32864198

Wang Y, Fardouly J, Vartanian LR, et al: Selfie-viewing and facial dissatisfaction among Chinese adolescents: a moderated mediation model of general attractiveness internalization and body appreciation. Body Image 30:35–43, 2019 31103791

Wilksch SM, O'Shea A, Ho P, et al: The relationship between social media use and disordered eating in young adolescents. Int J Eat Disord 53(1):96–106, 2020 31797420

Yau JC, Reich SM: "It's just a lot of work": adolescents' self-presentation norms and practices on Facebook and Instagram. J Res Adolesc 29(1):196–209, 2019 29430759

Zheng D, Ni X, Luo Y: Selfie posting on social networking sites and female adolescents' self-objectification: the moderating role of imaginary audience ideation. Sex Roles 80(5–6):325–331, 2019

12

Social Media, Self-Harm, and Suicide

Louise La Sala, Ph.D.

Eleanor Bailey, Ph.D.

Jo Robinson, Ph.D.

In this chapter, we encourage readers to consider both the opportunities and risks associated with social media and youth self-harm and suicide. Grounded in a theoretical model of suicidal behavior, we 1) provide an over-

---

Please note: For the purposes of this chapter, we mostly refer to *social media* as those platforms on which young people largely disclose their identity, interact with others via a profile/newsfeed, and are often held to account by those known to them in their offline lives (e.g., peers, friends and family, clinicians in the case of online interventions). The most popular platforms used by young people in Australia at this time fit these criteria and include Instagram, Snapchat, TikTok, Facebook, and Twitter/X. These differ from other online spaces, such as open-access forums or anonymous chat rooms. Although the affordances of social media slightly differ across each platform (e.g., some are more text-heavy, whereas others encourage the sharing of images), it is our hypothesis that young people specifically select certain online spaces to disclose information or share different parts of their mental health journey. Indeed, our most recent investigation into young people's motivations for using social media to communicate about self-harm indicated that young people predominantly use platforms with which they are already familiar to communicate about self-harm rather than seeking out apps or platforms to discuss self-harm or suicide (Thorn et al. 2023).

view of the types of self-harm- and suicide-related content to which young people may be exposed online; 2) introduce the #chatsafe guidelines and accompanying resources that have been used to support different youth populations; 3) discuss how social media can be used in clinical settings to support young people at risk of suicide; and 4) consider the implications of this use for both platforms and policymakers.

There is some contention in the literature over the definitions of *suicide*, *suicidal ideation*, and *self-harm* (Goodfellow et al. 2019). For the purposes of this chapter, we use the definitions recommended by De Leo et al. (2021; see Table 12–1). Although self-harm can occur without suicidal intent, we conceptualize self-harm as lying on a continuum of suicide and suicide-related behavior (i.e., not a distinct construct). This is because it is difficult to accurately identify the intention behind an episode of self-harm (e.g., due to challenges articulating intent or the fluctuation of intent) (Rasmussen et al. 2016). Moreover, suicide and self-harm share many of the same risk factors (Hawton et al. 2012), and self-harm, regardless of suicide intent, is the single-biggest risk factor for future suicide (Australian Institute of Health and Welfare 2023; Hawton et al. 2003). For these reasons, although we acknowledge that some differences between suicide- and self-harm-related social media use may exist, we have not attempted to distinguish between them in this chapter.

Rates of youth suicide and self-harm are increasing across the globe, with suicide the second leading cause of death among young people (World Health Organization 2019). When considering why youth self-harm and suicide rates remain high, many people have attempted to draw links between increasing rates of psychological distress experienced by young people and the amount of time they spend using social media. Although it is undisputed that social media has revolutionized the ways society, and in particular young people, communicate, it is far too simplistic to blame social media alone for a rise in youth self-harm and suicide. It is true that young people use social media to communicate about their distress and reach out for help, including to actively seek and receive information and support concerning self-harm and suicide in real time (Gibson and Trnka 2020; Lavis and Winter 2020; Nasier et al. 2021). It is also true that social media users could at times be exposed to unregulated, distressing, and potentially harmful content (Hawton et al. 2020; Yellow 2020). As we discuss in this chapter, in order to harness the benefits of online spaces while simultaneously mitigating the risks, it is important to critically engage with how young people use social media for the purposes of communicating about self-harm and

Table 12–1. Definitions of key terms

Suicide	An act resulting in death that is initiated and carried out by an individual to the end of the action, with the knowledge of a potentially fatal result, and in which intent may be ambiguous or unclear, may involve the risk of dying, or may not involve explicit intent to die
Suicidal ideation	To think of suicide with or without suicidal intent or hope for death by killing oneself, or to state suicidal intention without engaging in suicidal behavior
Self-harm	A nonfatal act in which a person harms themselves intentionally with varying motives, including the wish to die
Suicide attempt	An act in which a person harms themselves with the intention to die and survives

Source. Adapted from De Leo et al. 2021.

suicide and to codevelop solutions with young people for how they can keep themselves and their peers safe online.

A Theoretical Model of Suicide

One theory commonly used to understand suicidal behavior is the interpersonal theory of suicide (IPTS; Joiner 2005; Van Orden et al. 2010). This theory posits that suicide risk emerges when three psychological states exist simultaneously: perceived burdensomeness, thwarted belongingness, and acquired capability. *Perceived burdensomeness*, or the belief that one is a burden to others, comprises two dimensions: first, the belief that an individual's death is worth more to others than their life, and second, self-hate. *Thwarted belongingness* also comprises two dimensions: loneliness, or feeling disconnected from others, and lack of reciprocal care, or the feeling that one has nobody to turn to. Finally, *acquired capability* comprises a reduced fear of death and an elevated tolerance to physical and psychological pain. Taken together, these three simultaneous psychological states increase an individual's capacity for suicide and suicidal behavior.

The IPTS is relevant because social media may have the potential to both increase and ameliorate each of these factors (Bailey et al. 2018). For example, perceived burdensomeness may be increased by excessive exposure to the grief of others who have lost someone to suicide via memorial pages and sensationalist content; however, it may be reduced by the ability to support others while simultaneously receiving support oneself. Thwarted belongingness may be reduced by the sense of connection provided by supportive online communities. In contrast, acquired capability may be increased by exposure to detailed images or methods of self-harm or suicide. This theory has been applied in one small study (discussed in "A Clinical Example: Affinity" later in this chapter) that examined a therapeutic online social networking intervention with suicidal youth, with promising results (Bailey et al. 2020). However, to date, the IPTS has not been applied to population-wide campaigns designed to reduce risk of suicide or self-harm in youth.

Self-Harm- and Suicide-Related Content Online

Young people are known to use social media to communicate about self-harm and suicide in several ways. For example, they are known to discuss personal experiences with self-harm and suicide, to support their peers, and to communicate or share the news of a suicide death (Bailey et al. 2022; Gibson and Trnka 2020; Nasier et al. 2021; Robinson et al. 2016). Additionally, while some young people actively post or engage with this sort of content, it is not uncommon for others to be inadvertently exposed to self-harm- and suicide-related content posted by users (Arendt et al. 2019; Dunlop et al. 2011; Wakefield 2020). When it comes to assessing the safety of this content online, there is not a "one size fits all" approach for identifying content that is helpful or harmful for young people. Our work has suggested that what is deemed helpful by one young person may be considered unhelpful for someone else; furthermore, what is helpful for one individual at a particular point in time may also be unhelpful for them only moments later (Thorn et al. 2023). As a result, developing and providing guidance to youth, policy-makers, and the social media industry about what constitutes safe online communication about self-harm and suicide is both complex and nuanced.

Types of Content Young People View Online

We begin this section by discussing some of the potential harms associated with sharing suicide-related content on social media, then go on to describe some of the ways social media can be an important tool for support.

Online content relating to self-harm and suicide varies widely and includes images, photographs, videos, text, and combinations of these that are shared across multiple online spaces, for example, social media platforms, blogging websites, online news outlets, and online games. Not only does the type of content vary, but perceptions regarding what constitutes self-harm- and suicide-related content can also differ due to the range and diversity of content that relates to distress, sadness, loneliness, or hopelessness shared online by young people (Shanahan et al. 2019). This not only makes identifying self-harm- and suicide-related content difficult, it presents a real challenge when considering how social media users and social media companies should manage this type of content.

Although most social media platforms provide users with a range of safety features or community guidelines that prohibit the sharing of objectively unsafe content (e.g., live streams of suicide or graphic images relating to self-harm), many users, especially young people, establish ways of getting around these features. For example, young people are known to use cryptic or nondescript hashtags or search terms (e.g., "selfharn" instead of "self-harm") and to enter inaccurate dates of birth to bypass age restrictions for accessing certain types of content (Samaritans 2022). They are also more likely to move conversations to direct messages or more private groups. Despite users sometimes circumventing the safety functions, most of the literature supports the notion that the majority of self-harm- and suicide- related content shared by young people is intended to be helpful and often shared with good intentions (Brennan et al. 2022).

Regardless of whether the content is shared with good intentions or subjectively perceived to be helpful or harmful, many social media users consider themselves to have been exposed to self-harm- and suicide-related content online. A national survey conducted in the United Kingdom with individuals ages 16–84 years identified that 83% of their sample had been exposed to suicide-related content online, many before the age of 14 and mostly without intentionally searching for it (Samaritans 2022). Although not nationally representative samples, our own evaluations of youth-suicide-prevention social media campaigns echo these figures. In our first study, more than 50% of participants ages 16–25 ($N=189$; La Sala et al. 2021) reported seeing graphic descriptions of suicide, and more than a quarter had seen information about methods of suicide online. The second study recruited a sample of young people who had been exposed to the suicide or suicide attempt of someone they knew ($N=266$; La Sala et al. 2023), and more than a quarter of participants reported having seen suicide or goodbye notes, statements encouraging suicide, information regarding methods of suicide, and graphic descriptions of suicide online. Across both studies, around 30% of participants reported seeing statements that placed blame on others for someone else's safety or risk of suicide.

When young people are exposed to self-harm- or suicide-related content online, particularly if they know the person posting it, they likely feel a responsibility to respond or provide support. In a study exploring the impact of coronavirus disease 2019 (COVID-19) on young people's social media use (N=371; Bailey et al. 2022), 36% reported using social media to seek support for their own suicidal thoughts or self-harm, and more than 50% had provided online support to others. Of those who had supported others, 25% reported feeling worse after that interaction. Similarly, the U.K. study mentioned earlier in this section reported that viewing self-harm content on social media exacerbated participants' own distress and their urge to self-harm (Samaritans 2022), indicating that exposure to content and responding to content can be particularly difficult for young people, especially those with lived or living experience of self-harm and suicide.

Although the studies referred to here are from Australia and the United Kingdom, these data highlight the amount and nature of suicide-related content circulating online and its potential impact on some of the people who encounter it. The online context is not bound by geographical boundaries, and content can quickly move from one continent and platform to another. This means it is likely that young people across the globe are exposed to, and respond to, self-harm- and suicide-related content in a similar way.

Harms Associated With Exposure

One of the most-cited concerns about youth seeing self-harm- and suicide-related content online is *contagion*, the idea that viewing such information leads to an increase in suicide-related behavior. Similar to research in traditional media, a link has been identified between exposure to suicide-related content on social media and increases in suicidal thoughts, feelings, or behavior among young people (Arendt et al. 2019; Franklin et al. 2016; Samaritans 2022). Although this risk is higher when the information is shared in a particularly harmful or distressing way or when individuals overidentify (or closely identify) with the person experiencing suicidal distress, it is important to consider what role social media may play in encouraging imitative behavior, normalizing suicide, or increasing one's acquired capability.

Suicide clusters refers to a series of suicides that occur closer together within time and space than would be statistically expected (Hawton et al. 2020), and it is argued that clusters operate based on individuals being in close geographical, social, or psychological proximity to a suicide attempt or death. Given that exposure to suicide has been shown to increase subsequent risk among young people by around 300% (Hill et al. 2020), it is important to understand how exposure to suicide-related content on social media impacts young people. As stated earlier in "Types of Content Young People View Online," social media is not bound by geographical limitations, and individuals are connected globally. This reality redefines and expands our understanding of geographical, social, and psychological proximity. Social media not only increases the likelihood of young people being exposed to information about self-harm and suicide, it also increases the likelihood of them coming across individuals who experience suicidal distress or die from suicide. If we think about functionality and the speed at which content can be shared (e.g., live streaming), young people may well be exposed inadvertently to information about self-harm or suicide events, as well as to graphic depictions known to be distressing and harmful.

Although beyond the scope of this chapter, and often beyond that of the social media platforms considered here, we must be aware of online environments in which self-harm or suicide is glamorized and, at times, encouraged. For example, there are websites and forums that provide step-by-step information on methods of suicide (Dunlop et al. 2011). It is widely accepted that this type of communication is inherently harmful and more objectively contributes to one's acquired capability for suicide. As such, a lot of policy work across multiple jurisdictions globally has sought to remove these websites or prohibit them from being hosted in their respective regions.

To further counter these harms, many countries have developed or are developing legislation to regulate the types of content that can be shared online. Such approaches include the establishment of Australia's Office of the eSafety Commissioner to oversee the Online Safety Act; the 2013 amendment to the Children's Online Privacy Protection Act (COPPA) rule in the United States; and the Online Safety Bill in the United Kingdom. These efforts encourage social media companies to implement and enforce their own safety policies and terms of use, prohibiting or restricting access to a wide range of harmful content (for a more detailed overview of these safety functions, see Robinson et al. 2023, p. 121). However, policing or moderating these online and very global environments is difficult, if not impossible, suggesting that we need more than regulation alone to mitigate some of these harms. It also suggests that national legislation or platform-level policies can only go so far, and upskilling social media users with the digital literacy required to post and interact online in a safe way is equally important.

Benefits of Using Social Media to Communicate About Self-Harm and Suicide

Taking a different look at the argument posed earlier in this chapter, social media has reshaped the way we connect with others socially and psychologically and has broadened our social worlds much more than was previously possible. As such, we have more opportunities to meet like-minded others, access and receive immediate social support, and source high-quality and timely information. All of these aspects serve as protective factors for our mental health and highlight the beneficial and important role social media can play in a young person's life. Promoting a sense of connection and facilitating help-seeking in age-appropriate ways means social media has the potential to mitigate thwarted belongingness and perceived burdensomeness for young people who are struggling offline.

Our work, and that of many others, has shown that social media can provide an acceptable and accessible environment to seek help for and communicate about sensitive topics such as self-harm and suicide in a way that young people may feel unable to do offline (Brennan et al. 2022; Gibson and Trnka 2020; Robinson et al. 2016, 2017). This may be because they do not want to burden others with their problems or because self-harm and suicide are heavily stigmatized and difficult to discuss in the real world (Lavis and Winter 2020). Many youth also report negative experiences seeking help offline that make them less inclined to seek professional help and more inclined to turn to social media for support (Thorn et al. 2023). Youth with a lived or living experience of self-harm and suicide spend more time online, perhaps leading to (mis)interpreted claims of a causal link between social media and self-harm and suicide risk (Bailey et al. 2022). However, an alternative explanation is that these young people are likely getting the support or information they seek in an online environment, hence their desire to spend time on social media. Whatever the reason, social media appears to be an attractive, accessible, and age-appropriate way to seek information and support, particularly for sensitive or highly stigmatized topics.

Our research supports the notion that social media, when used carefully, can be a critical means of providing support and education to youth with regard to communicating about self-harm and suicide, knowing how to engage with such content, and assisting them in supporting others. We recently conducted a qualitative study in which we invited young people to share with us the harms and benefits of using social media to communicate about self-harm, including the motivations for having these conversations online. Although a running theme of these interviews was that what was helpful for one young person may not have been helpful for another young person or that same person at a different point in time, it was clear that social media was a source of important connection and often the only avenue for young people to communicate about their thoughts and practices of self-harm (Thorn et al. 2023). They explained that features such as anonymity, asynchronicity, and unlimited accessibility made this the case.

As noted, platform-based safety policies are one way of minimizing the harms of social media; however, this relies on the industry to self-regulate or respond to legislative policy actions. To fully capitalize on the benefits afforded by social media platforms, however, interventions are required that equip young people with the digital literacy to post and engage with social media content in a helpful way. Because different content has highly individualized impacts on different people, it is important to deliver psychoeducation to young people around helping them identify and navigate content that they find upsetting. Because young people sometimes prefer to seek information and support online, use social media to garner and provide support, and are increasingly reliant on these platforms for all elements of their social lives, equipping them with the tools to keep themselves and their peers safe online is a logical next step.

#chatsafe: Helping Young People Communicate Safely Online About Suicide and Self-Harm

In 2018, we created the #chatsafe guidelines to address concerns regarding youth using social media to talk about suicide (Robinson et al. 2018b). Developed via a Delphi consensus method, they were the world's first evidence-informed guidelines designed to support youth in communicating about suicide online safely. The #chatsafe guidelines comprise five sections (Figure 12–1) and were brought to life through a suicide prevention social media campaign (see www.instagram.com/chatsafe_au) designed in partnership with more than 130 young Australians. Delivered via Instagram, Snapchat, Facebook, Twitter, and Tumblr (Thorn et al. 2020), the guidelines reached 1.5 million young Australians in its first 3 months and has now reached more than 4 million young people worldwide (Robinson et al. 2021). In addition to the youth-facing campaign, the guidelines are also supported by a suite of adult-facing resources targeting parents and caregivers, educators and other school personnel, and local community/health organizations (see www.orygen.org.au/chatsafe).

> As young people, we want our support network to be well equipped with the understanding, skills, and resources so that they can support us. I feel more comfortable seeking help from those around me with the knowledge that they're being supported too.
>
> —*Ella, #chatsafe youth advisor*

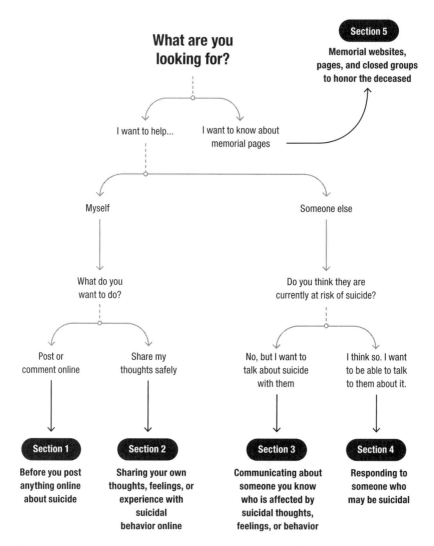

Figure 12–1. Structure and sections of the #chatsafe guidelines.

Recognizing the important role that social media can play in providing a sense of connection and reducing isolation, the #chatsafe intervention was not designed to reduce online communication about suicide but rather to enhance communication safety. It was evaluated in a general population sample of young people (*N*=189; La Sala et al. 2021) and then later in a sample of youth who had been exposed to a suicide or suicide attempt during the 2 years prior (*N*=266; La Sala et al. 2023). The aim of these studies was to examine the intervention's impact on the participants' confidence and capacity to communicate safely online about suicide, as well as their willingness to intervene after being exposed to online suicide-related content. Both studies saw improvements in these areas, as well as greater adherence to the recommendations of the #chatsafe guidelines. These results suggest that social media can be a safe and effective suicide prevention tool and that the #chatsafe intervention can decrease the harm associated with online communication about suicide. At this time, the #chatsafe intervention is being tested in a randomized controlled trial (trial ID: ACTRN12622001397707).

What Did Young People Think About the #chatsafe Social Media Campaign?

> Even though the topic of suicide is very sad, the content was never negative or too mournful…. I liked that a lot of the content were guidelines or things to think about instead of strict "rules." It got me thinking instead of just remembering what I'm supposed to say.
>
> *—anonymous participant*

> It makes me feel a lot more prepared and ready to handle a situation that involves suicide, which makes me feel that I can actually do something to change the situation.
>
> *—anonymous participant*

> It's helped me talk to teachers and well-being leaders about what we can do better to support those dealing with suicide and/or suicidal thoughts.
>
> *—anonymous participant*

> I lost someone really close to me to suicide, and this campaign made me feel more confident about discussing and talking about that.
>
> *—anonymous participant*

> I feel like I have gained a voice and am no longer afraid to speak of things that harmed me before.
>
> —*anonymous participant*

The following is an example of how the #chatsafe social media intervention is capitalizing on some of the benefits of social media and is being used as part of a real-time postvention response.

Using #chatsafe as a Real-Time Response to Youth Suicides in Australia

Young people who have been exposed to a suicide are at elevated risk (Hill et al. 2020), and communication about a suicide often occurs on social media. Hence, it is important to reach young people who have been exposed to a suicide in a timely manner with information about how to communicate safely about the death and how to seek help should they need it.

The #chatsafe intervention is capitalizing on the fact that social media can be used to reach targeted populations of young people with a suicide prevention intervention quickly and at relatively low cost. In partnership with local health departments, #chatsafe is now being used as a real-time response following the suicide of a young person in some parts of Australia (see Figure 12–2 for examples). Using targeted advertising, we disseminate a customized campaign that can be tailored for specific communities and target those people most likely to be impacted (e.g., school communities), based on their social or geographical proximity to the suicide.

To date, we have implemented more than 30 of these social media responses. The #chatsafe information is shared for 4–6 weeks in the form of two or three pieces of social media content that provide psychoeducation about suicide bereavement and include information on how to share news of a suicide safely and how to seek help. Together, these campaigns have reached almost 1 million social media users. Feedback from stakeholders within those communities has been that this approach was well received, has supported community members in safely communicating about suicide, and has encouraged help-seeking from local health services.

Working With Social Media in Clinical Practice

In this chapter we have described 1) the extent to which young people use social media, including to talk about self-harm and suicide; 2) motivations

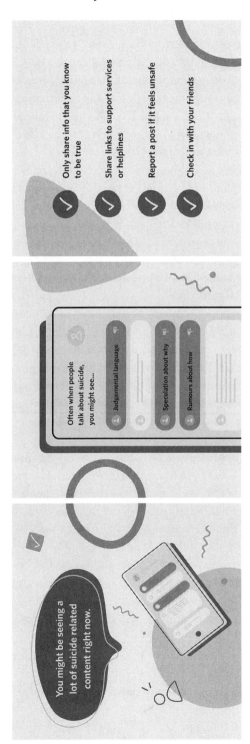

Figure 12–2. Examples of #chatsafe social media content that is used as a postvention response.

for using social media for this purpose (including help-seeking due to service gaps or negative experiences seeking help offline); and 3) the possible impacts, both positive and negative, that social media use can have on suicidal ideation and behavior. Thus, it is essential that professionals working with youth at risk of suicide remain cognizant of this and incorporate discussions about social media into their clinical practice. Discussions should occur collaboratively and in an ongoing way throughout a young person's episode of care. The aim of such discussions should not be to tell young people what they should and should not do online; rather, they should empower young people to be able to recognize and respond to the potential impacts (positive or negative) of their suicidal thoughts or behavior. Professionals should also be aware that young people will differ in whether and how social media influences their experience of self-harm or suicide, as well as whether and how they are affected by supporting someone else experiencing suicidal thoughts or self-harm and should take care not to make assumptions about the risks or benefits of their social media use.

Table 12–2 lists suggested prompts for helping professionals initiate conversations about social media and self-harm and suicide with young people. In general, they should explore how social media might *directly or indirectly* have a *positive or negative* impact on the youth's own thoughts about suicide or self-harm. They should also be mindful of the potential negative impact the young person's social media use might have on others and that the youth may not be aware of this impact. This should also be a focus of discussion, if relevant.

It is important for the helping professional to provide psychoeducation to the young person, as well as validate and normalize their experiences online (where appropriate). For example, some young people may struggle to recognize or acknowledge that providing support to a suicidal friend via social media is impacting them in a negative way and that they may need help from their clinician to build awareness of this and to manage it. Conversely, it is also important for clinicians to provide psychoeducation regarding how to manage any harmful or unsafe situations the young person may encounter and to escalate these appropriately, if needed (e.g., by seeking supervision or contacting authorities if concerned a young person may be encouraging self-harm or suicide online).

Once the professional and young person have a thorough understanding of the relationship between the youth's experience of suicidal thoughts or behavior and their social media use, consideration should be given to how this information may be used to minimize risks and maximize benefits in future. For example, if it is evident that a young person tends to withdraw from so-

Table 12–2. Prompts for helping professionals

What social media platforms do you use? How do you use them? (e.g., Do you post publicly, or do you mostly just look at other people's posts?)

What have you noticed about the way social media impacts your mood? Are there things you do or see online that are particularly helpful or unhelpful?

Do you ever see posts about suicide or self-harm on social media?

What kind of posts are they? What sorts of messages do they convey?

How does seeing these posts affect you? Do they ever make you feel more or less likely to act on your suicidal thoughts?

Do you ever post about your own suicidal thoughts or self-harm on social media?

What kinds of things do you post? Who would be able to see them?

What kind of response might you be hoping for?

Is posting about this helpful for you?

Do you think these posts might be helpful or harmful for the people who come across them?

In times when you have felt more suicidal (e.g., your thoughts or urges are more intense), does your social media use change? Tell me about this (e.g., different platforms, time spent online, ways platforms are used).

cial media when they are feeling suicidal, this could go into the "warning signs" section of a safety plan and be communicated to others who may notice this change in patterns and be able to intervene (e.g., friends or family members). Helping professionals should also educate young people about how to limit/filter content seen on social media, for example, by temporarily blocking potentially triggering accounts or setting time limits for social media access, as well as how to report or respond to content that is either unsafe for others or indicates a person may be at imminent risk of harm (for examples of how this can be done on social media platforms, see page 15 of the #chatsafe guidelines; Robinson et al. 2018a).

In addition to the important role helping professionals can play in educating and empowering young people, there is also scope for new treatment approaches/interventions that actively capitalize on the benefits afforded by social media to complement or extend the benefits of current clinical practice. The potential benefits of integrating digital tools into mental health care are well-documented and include their ability to provide around-the-clock support for little to no cost (Bucci et al. 2019a, 2019b; Knapp et al. 2021). However, given the risks associated with social media, professionally developed suicide prevention interventions have predominantly focused on static, self-guided formats and have failed to capitalize on social media's potential benefits. An exception to this is the Affinity intervention, described in the section that follows.

A Clinical Example: Affinity

Affinity is a website designed to be an adjunct to standard clinical care for young people experiencing suicidal ideation. It was developed and pilot-tested by a team of researchers at Orygen, a specialized youth mental health clinical and research facility in Melbourne, Australia, between 2018 and 2019. Affinity is based on the moderated online social therapy (MOST) model, which was initially designed for young people with early psychosis (Alvarez-Jimenez et al. 2013; Gleeson et al. 2012). The MOST model integrates three key components: peer-to-peer social networking, moderation by peer workers and clinicians, and therapeutic content delivered via comic-style content. At the time of this writing, Affinity is the first and only purpose-designed intervention for young people with suicidal ideation that specifically incorporates online peer-to-peer social networking.

The theoretical basis for Affinity drew heavily on the IPTS: specifically, we posited that the intervention's social networking component could increase belongingness (i.e., by providing access to a community of similar others) and reduce burdensomeness (i.e., via opportunities to support others) (Bailey et al. 2018). To mitigate the risks associated with social media (particularly the risk of contagion), a number of safety measures were put in place, including regular moderation of the social network and software that automatically blocked posts containing suicide-related keywords (i.e., effectively prohibiting posts or discussions about suicide on Affinity). In the pilot evaluation, Affinity was found to be safe, feasible, and acceptable (Bailey et al. 2020). Interviews with participants confirmed that they felt safe and experienced Affinity as a supportive environment; they also valued being a part of a network of similar others. They had mixed views about the safety measures: some felt better knowing they would not be exposed to suicide-related content on Affinity, whereas others felt they were censored and perceived this to increase the stigma around suicide (Bailey et al. 2021).

What Did Young People Think About Affinity?

People feel more secure being open in that area, as opposed to other social media. They could be attacked or feel triggered. But in Affinity, we're all here to support each other.

—*participant, age 22*

When I'm in a good mood, Facebook was great. But when I'm in a bad mood or have anxiety, I'm not sure, something about it upsets me. I never got that from Affinity. I'm not sure if it's because I didn't know the people, or it's because the posts were positive, or because I knew they were going through the same thing I was going through. Whatever it was, I never felt upset.

—*participant, age 23*

You read posts, and it would be something, you'd be like, oh, I've had that thought or that's how I feel. Then in your head you're like oh, this person's feeling that way too.... You read that post and think oh, okay, I'm not crazy, I'm not the only person that thinks that.

—*participant, age 22*

For me, it would be very triggering if I were to see anything about suicidal thoughts. But that depends on the person, I guess, because I think I'm just very emotional, and very easily influenced.

—*participant, age 23*

I know for myself sometimes when you want to…you just need to say something, and to some people it's going to sound really bad, but you're genuinely, like, I just need to get this out of my head.

—*participant, age 22*

Can Social Media Bridge the Gap Between Community and Clinical Approaches?

The Affinity example demonstrates how a social networking intervention can be effectively implemented in a clinical setting to deliver clinical care while also capitalizing on some of the benefits associated with social media, in particular by promoting connection and thereby mitigating the sense of thwarted belongingness associated with suicide risk. However, a key limitation remains in the sense that many young people experiencing suicide risk may not wish to seek help from, or be able to access, clinical services. Therefore, the question remains: can we use a social media–based intervention (such as #chatsafe) to help deliver evidence-based tools or interventions that both alleviate suicide risk and provide support to young people at risk in a way that does not rely on them coming forward to seek professional help?

When we have asked young people anecdotally if they think it would be acceptable to them to receive support via social media, their answer has been a resounding "yes." However, more research is required to understand: 1) if this type of intervention would be acceptable on a larger scale; 2) what interventions would be safe and appropriate to deliver in this way; and 3) how best to work in partnership with the social media industry to identify those young people who may be at risk. These questions are not straightforward to answer, and important ethical and safety considerations exist. Self-harm and suicide are complex and multifaceted problems that require solutions that are dynamic, nuanced, and age-appropriate—solutions in which social media could be a critical component.

Conclusion

In this chapter, we outlined the extent to which young people use social media to communicate about self-harm and suicide and what sort of content they are exposed to about these topics online. For many young people, there are clear motivations for turning to social media to communicate about self-harm and suicide, particularly if they are unable to seek appropriate help offline. For many others, exposure to information about self-harm and suicide is likely to be a part of their online interactions, with both positive and negative associated impacts. In this chapter, we identified #chatsafe as a case study for how social media could be used as an important tool to provide young people with suicide prevention information, and it has also highlighted important questions that helping professionals could ask when working with young people in a clinical setting.

We have also alluded to what some of the solutions could be. Given the complexity and nuance associated with the ways young people use social media to communicate about self-harm and suicide, and the dynamic nature of both suicidality and social media, these solutions will be multifaceted. In our view, solutions will need to include efforts on the part of the industry to develop and implement effective safety policies on their platforms, efforts to better equip youth with ways to keep themselves and their peers safe online, and efforts on the part of policymakers to integrate online safety into their suicide prevention strategies. Given the rising rates of self-harm and suicide among young people and their increasing use of social media in their day-to-day lives, it stands to reason that online safety needs to be a critical component of the suicide prevention landscape moving forward.

References

Alvarez-Jimenez M, Bendall S, Lederman R, et al: On the HORYZON: moderated online social therapy for long-term recovery in first episode psychosis. Schizophr Res 143(1):143–149, 2013 23146146

Arendt F, Scherr S, Romer D: Effects of exposure to self-harm on social media: evidence from a two-wave panel study among young adults. New Media Soc 21(11–12):2422–2442, 2019

Australian Institute of Health and Welfare: Psychosocial Risk Factors and Deaths by Suicide. Canberra, Australian Institute of Health and Welfare, 2023. Available at: https://www.aihw.gov.au/suicide-self-harm-monitoring/data/behaviours-risk-factors/psychosocial-risk-factors-suicide. Accessed December 5, 2023.

Bailey E, Rice S, Robinson J, et al: Theoretical and empirical foundations of a novel online social networking intervention for youth suicide prevention: a conceptual review. J Affect Disord 238:499–505, 2018 29936387

Bailey E, Alvarez-Jimenez M, Robinson J, et al: An enhanced social networking intervention for young people with active suicidal ideation: safety, feasibility, and acceptability outcomes. Int J Environ Res Public Health 17(7):2435, 2020 32260111

Bailey E, Robinson J, Alvarez-Jimenez M, et al: Moderated online social therapy for young people with active suicidal ideation: qualitative study. J Med Internet Res 23(4):e24260, 2021 33818392

Bailey E, Boland A, Bell I, et al: The mental health and social media use of young Australians during the COVID-19 pandemic. Int J Environ Res Public Health 19(3):1077, 2022 35162101

Brennan C, Saraiva S, Mitchell E, et al: Self-harm and suicidal content online, harmful or helpful? A systematic review of the recent evidence. J Public Ment Health 21(1):57–69, 2022

Bucci S, Berry N, Morris R, et al: "They are not hard-to-reach clients. We have just got hard-to-reach services." Staff views of digital health tools in specialist mental health services. Front Psychiatry 10:344, 2019a 31133906

Bucci S, Schwannauer M, Berry N: The digital revolution and its impact on mental health care. Psychol Psychother 92(2):277–297, 2019b 30924316

De Leo D, Goodfellow B, Silverman M, et al: International study of definitions of English-language terms for suicidal behaviours: a survey exploring preferred terminology. BMJ Open 11(2):e043409, 2021 33563622

Dunlop SM, More E, Romer D: Where do youth learn about suicides on the internet, and what influence does this have on suicidal ideation? J Child Psychol Psychiatry 52(10):1073–1080, 2011 21658185

Franklin JC, Fox KR, Franklin CR, et al: A brief mobile app reduces nonsuicidal and suicidal self-injury: evidence from three randomized controlled trials. J Consult Clin Psychol 84(6):544–557, 2016 27018530

Gibson K, Trnka S: Young people's priorities for support on social media: "It takes trust to talk about these issues." Comput Human Behav 102:238–247, 2020

Gleeson JF, Alvarez-Jimenez M, Lederman R: Moderated online social therapy for recovery from early psychosis. Psychiatr Serv 63(7):719, 2012 22752039

Goodfellow B, Kõlves K, de Leo D: Contemporary definitions of suicidal behaviour: a systematic literature review. Suicide Life Threat Behav 49(2):488–504, 2019 29574910

Hawton K, Zahl D, Weatherall R: Suicide following deliberate self-harm: long-term follow-up of patients who presented to a general hospital. Br J Psychiatry 182:537–542, 2003 12777346

Hawton K, Saunders KE, O'Connor RC: Self-harm and suicide in adolescents. Lancet 379(9834):2373–2382, 2012 22726518

Hawton K, Hill NTM, Gould M, et al: Clustering of suicides in children and adolescents. Lancet Child Adolesc Health 4(1):58–67, 2020 31606323

Hill NTM, Spittal MJ, Pirkis J, et al: Risk factors associated with suicide clusters in Australian youth: identifying who is at risk and the mechanisms associated with cluster membership. EClinicalMedicine 2930:100631, 2020 33294825

Joiner TE: Why People Die by Suicide. Cambridge, MA, Harvard University Press, 2005

Knapp AA, Cohen K, Nicholas J, et al: Integration of digital tools into community mental health care settings that serve young people: focus group study. JMIR Ment Health 8(8):e27379, 2021 34420928

La Sala L, Teh Z, Lamblin M, et al: Can a social media intervention improve online communication about suicide? A feasibility study examining the acceptability and potential impact of the #chatsafe campaign. PLoS One 16(6):e0253278, 2021 34129610

La Sala L, Pirkis J, Cooper C, et al: Acceptability and potential impact of the #chatsafe suicide postvention response among young people who have been exposed to suicide: pilot study. JMIR Human Factors 10:e44535, 2023 37204854

Lavis A, Winter R: #Online harms or benefits? An ethnographic analysis of the positives and negatives of peer-support around self-harm on social media. J Child Psychol Psychiatry 61(8):842–854, 2020 32459004

Nasier B, Gibson K, Trnka S: "PM me" or "LOL": young peoples' observations of supportive and unsympathetic responses to distress on social media. Comput Human Behav 124:106933, 2021

Rasmussen S, Hawton K, Philpott-Morgan S, et al: Why do adolescents self-harm? An investigation of motives in a community sample. Crisis 37(3):176–183, 2016 26831210

Robinson J, Cox G, Bailey E, et al: Social media and suicide prevention: a systematic review. Early Interv Psychiatry 10(2):103–121, 2016 25702826

Robinson J, Bailey E, Hetrick S, et al: Developing social media-based suicide prevention messages in partnership with young people: exploratory study. JMIR Ment Health 4(4):e40, 2017 28978499

Robinson J, Hill NTM, Thorn P, et al: #chatsafe: A Young Person's Guide for Communicating Safely Online About Suicide. Parkville, Australia, Orygen, 2018a. Available at: https://www.orygen.org.au/chatsafe. Accessed December 5, 2023.

Robinson J, Hill NTM, Thorn P, et al: The #chatsafe project: developing guidelines to help young people communicate safely about suicide on social media: a Delphi study. PLoS One 13(11):e0206584, 2018b 30439958

Robinson J, Teh Z, Lamblin M, et al: Globalization of the #chatsafe guidelines: using social media for youth suicide prevention. Early Interv Psychiatry 15(5):1409–1413, 2021 32935440

Robinson J, La Sala L, Battersby-Coulter R: Safely navigating the terrain: keeping young people safe online, in Social Media and Mental Health. Edited by Brennan C, House A. New York, Cambridge University Press, 2023, pp 121–130

Samaritans: How social media users experience self-harm and suicide content. Samaritans, November 8, 2022. Available at: https://www.samaritans.org/news/samaritans-report-reveals-dangers-of-social-medias-self-harm-content. Accessed December 5, 2023.

Shanahan N, Brennan C, House A: Self-harm and social media: thematic analysis of images posted on three social media sites. BMJ Open 9(2):e027006, 2019 30782950

Thorn P, Hill NT, Lamblin M, et al: Developing a suicide prevention social media campaign with young people (the #chatsafe project): co-design approach. JMIR Ment Health 7(5):e17520, 2020 32391800

Thorn P, La Sala L, Hetrick S, et al: Motivations and perceived harms and benefits of online communication about self-harm: an interview study with young people. Digit Health 9:20552076231176689, 2023 37252260

Van Orden KA, Witte TK, Cukrowicz KC, et al: The interpersonal theory of suicide. Psychol Rev 117(2):575–600, 2010 20438238

Wakefield J: TikTok tries to remove widely shared suicide clip. BBC News, September 8, 2020. Available at: https://www.bbc.com/news/technology-54069650. Accessed December 5, 2023.

World Health Organization: Suicide Worldwide in 2019. Geneva, World Health Organization, 2019. Available at: https://www.who.int/publications/i/item/9789240026643. Accessed December 5, 2023.

Yellow: Yellow Social Media Report 2020: Part One—Consumers. 2020. Available at: https://sensis.wpenginepowered.com/wp-content/uploads/sites/2/2020/07/Yellow-Social-Media-Report-2020-Consumer-Statistics.pdf. Accessed December 5, 2023.

13

Role of Social Media Applications in Clinical Treatment

Justine Bautista, M.A.
Stephen M. Schueller, Ph.D.
Kaylee P. Kruzan, Ph.D., L.S.W.

In this chapter, we delve into the exciting possibilities of integrating social media into clinical mental health interventions for young people. Specifically, we explore different ways social media can play a role in clinical applications, including as a conduit for content dissemination and psychoeducation and as a component of digital intervention. We also explore the qualities of social media that are most conducive to mental health intervention. Finally, we highlight the challenges and considerations that must be addressed when using social media in a clinical context.

Nearly half of all teenagers have indicated that they use social media almost constantly (Vogels et al. 2022). The rise of social media use has paralleled a youth mental health crisis in the United States. As such, considerable research has been done and investment made in understanding the risks associated with social media (Karim et al. 2020) and finding ways to leverage its qualities within mental health intervention (e.g., digital mental health applications [apps]) to provide support to teenagers in need (Shah and Berry 2020; Wind et al. 2020). This provides an unprecedented opportunity to deliver mental health resources that meet adolescents where they are.

We define *social media* as any internet-based communication platform or app that enables interaction between users, especially the sharing or consuming of information. *Social media intervention* is a broad term that we have adopted to describe the use of social media features and functionalities to improve clinical mental health outcomes. This means social media interventions come in different shapes and sizes. In this chapter, we focus on the use of social media 1) as a platform for information delivery and dissemination, 2) to distribute evidence-based clinical interventions, and 3) as a component of a digital intervention (e.g., mobile app, Web-based). We also note opportunities for social media data to be used to improve and enhance clinical care by gaining a better understanding of patients' experiences through machine learning/artificial intelligence (AI) on existing social media platforms (e.g., Instagram, TikTok) or new platforms developed specifically for an intervention (Radovic et al. 2022). Integrating social media into clinical intervention means either incorporating existing social media content, such as psychoeducation materials, into a patient's clinical treatment or designing and developing an intervention for delivery through social media.

Digital interventions are relevant across a continuum of care opportunities. For example, the integration of machine learning and AI with social media data has shown promising results for the improvement of clinical care and decision-making (Su et al. 2020). In the area of prevention for low-intensity needs, social media can play a role in providing psychoeducation and peer stories. Furthermore, for patients who have low-intensity needs or are waiting for treatment, social media can provide basic skills training, empowering them to manage their health more effectively. It may also be used to provide adjunctive resources during formal care, such as the use of apps that offer peer support groups, enabling patients to connect with others going through similar experiences. Different uses of social media across the continuum of care are explicated in Figure 13–1.

Opportunities of Social Media Interventions

Social Media for Psychoeducation

I usually ask my friends what mental [health] apps they use or see what is trending on social media.

—*Ashley, age 20*

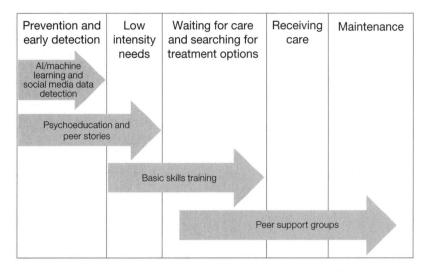

Figure 13–1. Social media across the continuum of care.

Social media is frequently used to access health and mental health information and to connect with similar people for advice related to mental health issues. Youth often turn to social media and to their peers when deciding which interventions to engage in. In recent years, the widespread use of social media has transformed it into a public health resource, allowing both users and professionals to send and spread mental health information, often through campaigns that can serve as prevention and intervention tools reaching a large and diverse audience. Psychoeducation is especially valuable in earlier stages of the continuum of care, providing initial information to identify and assess mental health needs and, in cases in which the information is peer-generated and non-evidence-based, offering many opportunities for destigmatization.

Peer-Provided Content

One study evaluated the impact of an Instagram-based outreach campaign to increase engagement, retention, awareness, and quality of experiences in a cohort of adolescents (Thomas et al. 2020). The campaign involved creating an Instagram account that consisted of codesigned mental health content. This appeared to increase the engagement and retention of participants for their intervention study, signaling a particular interest in social media–delivered psychoeducation for adolescents. The following are examples of peer-generated content, some of them participating in platform campaigns:

- Dear My Anxiety (@dearmyanxiety) on Instagram was created by mental health advocate Stefania Rossi and provides daily posts about anxiety, including self-care tips. As of 2024, the account had amassed more than 350,000 followers.
- "Hi Anxiety" is a digital campaign featuring celebrities who share their mental health stories; as of 2024, the campaign has 170,000 followers (www.hianxiety.org).
- "Seize the Awkward" is a similar digital campaign in which celebrities and influencers discuss mental health and provide information regarding how to support others (https://seizetheawkward.org). The campaign has reached more than 30,000 followers.
- With the "Egg" campaign, which featured a brown egg and aimed to set the record for the most likes on a single Instagram post (Gionfriddo and Reinert 2019), viewers were encouraged to visit Mental Health America for online screening. Within one day of the campaign, more than 5,000 people had visited the screening site (Gionfriddo and Reinert 2019).

Although some of these campaigns are no longer active, and engagement with specific social media accounts may fluctuate, new initiatives and innovations are always emerging. Social media is a rapidly growing and changing realm, but its exponential popularity among youth seems to be the constant amid all the changes. They continue to engage with social media and digital campaigns to address mental health themselves.

Expert-Generated Content

Expert-generated content refers to materials created by mental health professionals or other experts on social media. Ideally, this type of content provides users with evidence-based, accurate information about mental health. Examples include

- A medical-education talk show available on YouTube featuring a board-certified psychologist and advertised to Chinese-speaking individuals; results from a study by Lam and Woo (2020) found that about two-thirds of this show's views came from Instagram.
- Dr. Julie Smith (@drjulie) on TikTok had amassed nearly 5 million followers by January 2024 and tackles a number of mental health conditions, providing informational videos and strategies for coping.

Blended Expert- and Peer-Provided Content

Social media also offers opportunities for blended expert and peer-generated support. Examples include

- The Mental Health Coalition's *Every Day in May: 1-2-1 Series,* which features a discussion between an influencer and an advocate around a specific mental health topic via Instagram each day (The Mental Health Coalition 2021)
- Supporting Our Valued Adolescents (SOVA), a social media website featuring both expert-generated psychoeducation materials and moderated user posts (Radovic et al. 2018)

Digital Applications for Mental Health

The marketplace of mental health apps is vast and growing. The thousands of available apps represent considerable variation in quality and effectiveness. Although some have integrated science-backed interventions or been evaluated in clinical research demonstrating their usefulness and effectiveness, most have no research evidence whatsoever (Neary and Schueller 2018). Analyses of the features of mental health apps have often found that the majority consist of the same foundational elements, the most common of which being psychoeducation, goal setting, mindfulness, and tracking (Camacho et al. 2022). Perhaps most relevant to this chapter, some apps allow connections with others to provide peer support, but despite the general allure of social apps, this is a relatively less common feature.

Very few mental health apps are targeted specifically toward teenagers, despite this population's noted desire for apps that specifically address the challenges they face (Agapie et al. 2022). Generally, the research that has been conducted on mental health apps for children and adolescents has found that they can be effective, but such studies are often small pilot or feasibility studies that do not examine long-term outcomes (Grist et al. 2017). Despite the lack of evidence, however, many adolescents are turning to mental health apps to find support. A recent survey of 14- to 22-year-olds found that 61% had used a mobile app related to health; this number grew to 75% among those with moderate to severe depressive symptoms (Rideout et al. 2021). Many of the apps these youth reported using were related to mental health concerns, including sleep, mindfulness, stress reduction, mood, and depression. While their use of interventions may not be consistent, youth seem to engage in interventions quite frequently.

I indirectly use [mental health apps] every day. I don't have a routine, it's by chance that I see it, which in my opinion, makes it more fun!

—anonymous teen

Usually, I use it under extreme circumstances, like before a performance or presentation. I want to be able to implement it in my everyday routine in the future.

—Ashley, age 20

Mental health apps can also be used as an adjunct to professional mental health care. For example, they can be used in conjunction with therapy to provide additional support and resources between sessions. In addition to helping users self-manage by increasing their knowledge and practicing skills, app data can be invaluable for clinicians because they can be used to track symptoms and monitor progress, which can provide valuable information for treatment.

Properties of Social Media for Mental Health Care

Social media interventions have demonstrated preliminary efficacy in improving mental health outcomes (Kruzan et al. 2022), although they have yet to be widely deployed. However, insights from current research suggest that such interventions can be used across the entire continuum of care, providing low-intensity and scalable support or resources for prevention and early intervention and acting as a supplement to traditional care. Benefits include reducing stigma and enhancing peer-to-peer connections (Alonzo and Popescu 2021; Coulson and Buchanan 2022; Naslund et al. 2016). Social media interventions can also provide clinicians with invaluable data to enhance their clinical understanding of patient mental health. Data from Twitter have been used to predict patterns of depression, allowing us to better understand population-level trends (De Choudhury et al. 2014).

Personalization

One attractive characteristic of social media interventions is the ability to personalize and customize participant experiences. This can be accomplished through various social media features, such as messages, content, and conversations. For example, Momentum is an app and online social network that provides therapy modules and features 12 mindfulness-based steps aimed at promoting well-being (Alvarez-Jimenez et al. 2018). This intervention uses expert moderation to send tailored content and messages based on the participant's needs, strengths, and interests, which has led to elevated levels of engagement, social functioning, and subjective well-being.

Peer Support Versus Stigma

Interventions that integrate peer support through social media allow participants to engage with others facing similar challenges. By having conversations openly with peers online, people can break through the stigma around mental health. For example, in online support groups for people affected by HIV and AIDS, members reported reduced stigma and improved self-worth (Coulson and Buchanan 2022). Although many traditional interventions involve sparse contact with one or several individuals, social media facilitates open discussion and engagement with a broader social network, which may empower participants to address self-stigma and experience improved outcomes. We interviewed one teenager who spoke about the benefits that online spaces provided during college admissions season:

> During college applications, it's very easy to feel alone or stressed out. As an only child, I didn't feel like many understood. There are many high school dedicated spaces that allow seniors to relate and share advice more freely and less competitively online.
>
> *—anonymous teen*

The anonymity provided by many social media platforms presents an opportunity for individuals who may not otherwise participate in face-to-face discussions regarding mental health to engage in online conversations. Anonymous participation may reduce social judgment and the risks associated with disclosure of mental health issues (Thomas et al. 2015). This network of people may also be especially useful for those who feel socially isolated. For example, an Asian individual in a predominantly White community may experience high mental health stigma and may not feel comfortable disclosing information to others in their immediate environment. Engaging with peers through an online social media intervention allows the person to communicate with others who understand their unique background and the stigma associated with it.

Engagement and Attrition

Engagement and attrition are prominent concerns in care delivery that social media interventions may address. Building clinical interventions into existing social media platforms leverages these networks for reach and engagement while promoting a sense of mutual support, which may ultimately lead to better engagement and less attrition (Alvarez-Jimenez et al. 2014). Delivery of interventions through social media may also overcome some of the accessibility challenges of traditional in-person interventions. Participants can access interventions in their own homes and on their own time, cutting down travel costs and scheduling.

Cost and Availability

> I would look mainly for accessibility [no cost]...
>
> —*anonymous teen*

For youth, accessibility of an intervention is at the forefront of their concerns, and digital interventions can provide an accessible option for support. In an economic evaluation of cognitive-behavioral therapy (CBT) delivered via the internet or in person, integration of the internet-delivered component reduced cost of care without diminishing efficacy (Aspvall et al. 2021). Those who used the internet-delivered intervention also used fewer therapist resources, minimizing the burden on a health care system that is already stretched thin. Furthermore, social media interventions are always available, allowing patients to access care immediately and when a clinician may not be readily available.

Challenges and Considerations

Using social media interventions to improve clinical outcomes has great potential to reach a wide audience and to engage them in their own mental health care. Their implementation is a multifaceted and challenging endeavor requiring careful consideration of numerous limitations. Challenges may include 1) understanding the impact and effect of the intervention, 2) inequality in access to technology, known as the "digital divide," that affects certain populations' ability to access social media and social media interventions, 3) the potential for digital overload, in which users may be overwhelmed by the volume of information on the internet and experience difficulty maintaining their attention, 4) misinformation challenges, such as distinguishing between false and valid claims on social media sites, and

5) safety and privacy concerns associated with sharing personal information online, especially in light of data breaches and online harassment.

Understanding the Impact

Social media encompasses multiple platforms, each with myriad features, a multitude of users, and, for popular platforms, a massive amount of content. As such, it is not a monolithic entity. Certain aspects or uses might be effective, whereas others might not, and some might even be harmful. Behavioral outcomes from app use may vary greatly according to individual differences such as the user's psychosocial makeup, level of engagement, goal setting, and intensity of use (Zhang et al. 2019). As a result, it is likely that different ways of engaging with social media interventions may also have different outcomes. In particular, frequent exposure to idealized versions of peers on social media can lead to negative outcomes such as body dissatisfaction (Kleemans et al. 2018). Exposure to age-inappropriate content such as violence, sexual content, and hate speech is also a challenge for young people using social media (Livingstone and Helsper 2008).

One Mind PsyberGuide (https://adaa.org/psyberguide) provided a credibility rating system for mental health apps based on several metrics, including user experience, credibility, and transparency, and offered a professional review along with recommendations for use (Neary et al. 2021). The One Mind PsyberGuide project was funded through May 2023, and all resources reviewed on the website include a date indicating when the review was completed. Other organizations also provide information about mental health apps, including the Anxiety and Depression Association of America, the M-health Index and Navigation Database (MIND Apps), and the Mozilla Foundation. Challenges in understanding the impact of various apps include a rapidly changing social media landscape and the individual user's context, making it important to focus on features and functions rather than platforms. Although traditional social media platforms are used regularly in people's daily lives, the context and manner in which people interact with social media vary widely, making it difficult to separate the effect of a specific social media intervention from other general social media use and environmental factors.

Most examples of current social media interventions are multicomponent, making it difficult to determine which component elicited an outcome (Laranjo et al. 2015). Social media itself is often multifaceted, delivering content while simultaneously offering users several different ways to engage with the content and with each other. Social media interventions have only recently begun to be studied, so standardized methods of exploring its effects are lacking, and little clinical validation for existing interventions is yet available (Attai et al. 2016). Moreover, platforms are continuously evolving, making it increasingly difficult to create and validate new methods.

The Digital Divides

Several factors can make the consistent application of social media in clinical practice challenging, including generational, socioeconomic, and geographical differences. Generational gaps exist in people's use and exposure to technology, shaping their expectations and knowledge. Age and period of life shape people's platform preferences and the relevance of social media campaigns and online content. This makes it especially important to consider the targeted end-user because each may have different preferences for, comfort with, and understanding of social media. To this end, research has shown that end-users are far more likely to prefer an intervention delivered through a device that is familiar to them (Granger et al. 2016).

Access to Wi-Fi and a stable internet connection are required for virtually all social media platforms and may be lacking in many rural communities. Although social media use is pervasive across socioeconomic status (SES) and geography, the stability with which individuals can access and engage with all features varies. Some may have difficulty accessing a video if their home Wi-Fi does not possess the necessary bandwidth. SES and education level are significant predictors of digital intervention use, indicating that people of lower SES and lower education level are less likely to engage in social media interventions (Kontos et al. 2014). Issues of poverty, costs associated with access, and broadband availability in areas with higher concentrations of rural, lower SES households may affect youth's access to digital interventions (Reddick et al. 2020).

Skill building along with mental health literacy and digital literacy are central to digital intervention access (Ramakrishnan et al. 2022; Zheng and Walsham 2021). Lower-SES youth report higher occurrences of negative online experiences and poorer psychological well-being (George et al. 2020). Furthermore, among Indigenous youth, technological barriers (e.g., screen freezing, bandwidth when other family members are also using devices) were the most commonly cited concerns when accessing electronic health (eHealth) interventions (Toombs et al. 2021). Black and Hispanic individuals in rural communities are also less likely to have reliable access to the internet (Choi et al. 2022). Thus, with the increasing availability and use of social media interventions, it is imperative to understand issues of intersectionality and how these interventions can be more inclusive.

Overload and Misinformation

As social media sites expand their features and user bases, the amount of content available on these platforms also expands—often exponentially—leading to the potential for information overload. This increasing volume, combined with platform business models fed by customization and recommendation algorithms, may make it difficult for users to identify misleading content, perpetuating misinformation (Guilbeault et al. 2018). Users may become siloed into echo chambers of information and, along with it, misinformation. Information overload and misinformation are especially relevant to content sharing for clinical purposes. The quality of the content is not related to increased views and engagement, suggesting that poor-quality content is as likely as high-quality content to reach the masses (Qiu et al. 2017), and overload remains a concern as users fail to keep up with social media content tailored to them (Park 2019).

The spread of health-related misinformation has grown increasingly prevalent in recent years. Although the sharing of user-generated content with others is a strength of social media platforms, not all of this content is accurate, and inaccurate information can lead to wide dissemination of misinformation. Youth desire peer-to-peer support that is professionally moderated to ensure their safety (Aschbrenner et al. 2019); yet, to moderate and deliver the intervention effectively in real time, interventionists must be available during off-hours (Pagoto et al. 2016). Moderation is a major challenge because neither manual human moderation nor automated technological moderation are sufficient to detect all instances of inaccurate or harmful content (Gongane et al. 2022).

Safety and Privacy Concerns

For clinicians, social media may present privacy and safety risks, such as blurred authority and boundaries in therapeutic relationships, because patients may be able to find and contact providers outside of the treatment environment. Privacy breaches are most likely for providers who have higher online presences (Kaluzeviciute 2020). Privacy and security issues also are prominent concerns for youth (Robinson et al. 2016; Saberi et al. 2016); they have cited concerns with security and stigma and fears around how data breaches and personal information leaks may affect the perception of their peers toward them (Saberi et al. 2016). However, private and moderated social media interventions designed or adapted specifically for clinical practice are possible and can provide a valuable safe space for youth (Gleeson et al. 2014). Large, multipurpose social media platforms (e.g., Facebook, Instagram) have been used to deliver mental health interventions but were not designed to facilitate the exchange of mental health support. As a result, they may lack the privacy and security features (including things such as anonymity) of purpose-built mental health apps designed to provide a confidential and private environment for sharing mental health information.

Conclusion and Future Directions

Clinical social media interventions are relatively new, and innovative thinking is needed to address the challenges described here. Interdisciplinary academic-industry collaborations could be especially beneficial in creating such interventions (Kruzan et al. 2022). Some challenges that social media interventions face may require partnerships with policymakers and additional stakeholders to address, such as improving infrastructure and increasing access to technology by specific populations and geographical areas, especially rural areas. Partnerships between industry and government stakeholders could also allow researchers and clinicians to advocate for privacy and security standards while holding social media platforms accountable when privacy breaches occur. In addition, engaging consumers, and especially youth, in both the evaluation and development of interventions can provide valuable insights into how they engage with the interventions, what elements of an intervention are effective (or ineffective) for them, and how the intervention can be tailored to them.

Clinicians can use social media content in their treatment sessions to educate and engage their patients. Content from social media posts can provide visual aids and mental health topics to better understand concepts being discussed in therapy, which may be especially useful for youth by providing a more relatable and approachable way to discuss mental health. Creating a more interactive and engaging session may be especially beneficial for youth who struggle to engage in conversations about their mental health and may enhance the patient-provider relationship, making it easier to connect and to understand the information shared.

Mental health stigma is a prominent barrier to help-seeking, and effective social media interventions can provide support that reduces stigma and provides patients with anonymous, confidential care (Robinson et al. 2016). However, ensuring that these interventions reduce stigma requires careful consideration of the content to ensure it also does not cause harm. In one social media campaign study, for example, stigmatizing content had the most engagement in terms of retweets and favorites on Twitter (Saha et al. 2019). In light of this, it is worth noting that many of the potential benefits of social media will only be realized if it is used thoughtfully. Cross-sector partnerships between academia, industry, nonprofits, and content creators will likely be necessary to ensure that social media messages reduce, rather than exacerbate, mental health stigma.

References

Agapie E, Chang K, Patrachari S, et al: Understanding mental health apps for youth: focus group study with Latinx youth. JMIR Form Res 6(10):e40726, 2022 36256835

Alonzo D, Popescu M: Utilizing social media platforms to promote mental health awareness and help seeking in underserved communities during the COVID-19 pandemic. J Educ Health Promot 10(1):156, 2021 34222531

Alvarez-Jimenez M, Alcázar-Córcoles MÁ, González-Blanch C, et al: Online, social media and mobile technologies for psychosis treatment: a systematic review on novel user-led interventions. Schizophr Res 156(1):96–106, 2014 24746468

Alvarez-Jimenez M, Gleeson JF, Bendall S, et al: Enhancing social functioning in young people at ultra high risk (UHR) for psychosis: a pilot study of a novel strengths and mindfulness-based online social therapy. Schizophr Res 202(December):369–377, 2018 30031616

Aschbrenner KA, Naslund JA, Tomlinson EF, et al: Adolescents' use of digital technologies and preferences for mobile health coaching in public mental health settings. Front Public Health 7:178, 2019 31312629

Aspvall K, Sampaio F, Lenhard F, et al: Cost-effectiveness of internet-delivered vs in-person cognitive behavioral therapy for children and adolescents with obsessive-compulsive disorder. JAMA Netw Open 4(7):e2118516, 2021 34328501

Attai DJ, Sedrak MS, Katz MS, et al: Social media in cancer care: highlights, challenges and opportunities. Future Oncol 12(13):1549–1552, 2016 27025657

Camacho E, Cohen A, Torous J: Assessment of mental health services available through smartphone apps. JAMA Netw Open 5(12):e2248784, 2022 36576737

Choi EY, Kanthawala S, Kim YS, et al: Urban/rural digital divide exists in older adults: does it vary by racial/ethnic groups? J Appl Gerontol 41(5):1348–1356, 2022 35196918

Coulson NS, Buchanan H: The role of online support groups in helping individuals affected by HIV and AIDS: scoping review of the literature. J Med Internet Res 24(7):e27648, 2022 35881456

De Choudhury M, Counts SE, Horvitz E, et al: Characterizing and predicting postpartum depression from shared Facebook data, in CHI'14: Proceedings of the 17th ACM Conference on Computer Supported Cooperative Work and Social Computing. New York, Association for Computing Machinery, 2014, pp 626–638

George MJ, Jensen MR, Russell MA, et al: Young adolescents' digital technology use, perceived impairments, and well-being in a representative sample. J Pediatr 219(April):180–187, 2020 32057438

Gionfriddo P, Reinert M: Why the egg matters. Mental Health America, 2019. Available at: https://mhanational.org/blog/why-egg-matters. Accessed December 5, 2023.

Gleeson JF, Lederman R, Wadley G, et al: Safety and privacy outcomes from a moderated online social therapy for young people with first-episode psychosis. Psychiatr Serv 65(4):546–550, 2014 24687106

Gongane VU, Munot MV, Anuse AD: Detection and moderation of detrimental content on social media platforms: current status and future directions. Soc Netw Anal Min 12(1):129, 2022 36090695

Granger D, Vandelanotte C, Duncan MJ, et al: Is preference for mHealth intervention delivery platform associated with delivery platform familiarity? BMC Public Health 16(1):619, 2016 27450240

Grist R, Porter J, Stallard P: Mental health mobile apps for preadolescents and adolescents: a systematic review. J Med Internet Res 19(5):e176, 2017 28546138

Guilbeault D, Becker J, Centola D: Social learning and partisan bias in the interpretation of climate trends. Proc Natl Acad Sci USA 115(39):9714–9719, 2018 30181271

Kaluzeviciute G: Social media and its impact on therapeutic relationships. Br J Psychother 36(2):303–320, 2020

Karim F, Oyewande AA, Abdalla LF, et al: Social media use and its connection to mental health: a systematic review. Cureus 12(6):e8627, 2020 32685296

Kleemans M, Daalmans S, Carbaat I, et al: Picture perfect: the direct effect of manipulated Instagram photos on body image in adolescent girls. Media Psychol 21(1):93–110, 2018

Kontos E, Blake KD, Chou W-YS, et al: Predictors of eHealth usage: insights on the digital divide from the Health Information National Trends Survey 2012. J Med Internet Res 16(7):e172, 2014 25048379

Kruzan KP, Williams KDA, Meyerhoff J, et al: Social media-based interventions for adolescent and young adult mental health: a scoping review. Internet Interv 30:100578, 2022 36204674

Lam NHT, Woo BKP: Efficacy of Instagram in promoting psychoeducation in the Chinese-speaking population. Health Equity 4(1):114–116, 2020 32258963

Laranjo L, Arguel A, Neves AL, et al: The influence of social networking sites on health behavior change: a systematic review and meta-analysis. J Am Med Inform Assoc 22(1):243–256, 2015 25005606

Livingstone S, Helsper E: Parental mediation of children's internet use. J Broadcast Electron Media 52(4):581–599, 2008

Mental Health Coalition: Every day in May: 121 series. Mental Health Coalition, May 4, 2021. Available at: https://www.thementalhealthcoalition.org/121-series. Accessed December 6, 2023.

Naslund JA, Aschbrenner KA, Marsch LA, et al: The future of mental health care: peer-to-peer support and social media. Epidemiol Psychiatr Sci 25(2):113–122, 2016 26744309

Neary M, Schueller SM: State of the field of mental health apps. Cogn Behav Pract 25(4):531–537, 2018 33100810

Neary M, Bunyi J, Palomares K, et al: A process for reviewing mental health apps: using the One Mind PsyberGuide credibility rating system. Digit Health 7:20552076211053690, 2021 34733541

Pagoto S, Waring ME, May CN, et al: Adapting behavioral interventions for social media delivery. J Med Internet Res 18(1):e24, 2016 26825969

Park CG: Does too much news on social media discourage news seeking? Mediating role of news efficacy between perceived news overload and news avoidance on social media. Soc Media Soc 5(3):1–12, 2019

Qiu X, Oliveira DFM, Shirazi AS, et al: Limited individual attention and online virality of low-quality information. Nat Hum Behav 1(7), 2017

Radovic A, Gmelin T, Hua J, et al: Supporting Our Valued Adolescents (SOVA), a social media website for adolescents with depression and/or anxiety: technological feasibility, usability, and acceptability study. JMIR Ment Health 5(1):e17, 2018 29483067

Radovic A, Li Y, Landsittel D, et al: A social media website (Supporting Our Valued Adolescents) to support treatment uptake for adolescents with depression or anxiety: pilot randomized controlled trial. JMIR Ment Health 9(10):e35313, 2022 36206044

Ramakrishnan T, Ngamassi L, Rahman S: Examining the factors that influence the use of social media for disaster management by underserved communities. Int J Disaster Risk Sci 13(1):52–65, 2022

Reddick CG, Enriquez R, Harris RJ, et al: Determinants of broadband access and affordability: an analysis of a community survey on the digital divide. Cities 106:102904, 2020 32921864

Rideout V, Fox S, Peebles A, et al: Coping With COVID-19: How Young People Use Digital Media to Manage Their Mental Health. Common Sense Media, 2021. Available at: https://www.commonsensemedia.org/research/coping-with-covid-19-how-young-people-use-digital-media-to-manage-their-mental-health. Accessed November 30, 2023.

Robinson J, Cox G, Bailey E, et al: Social media and suicide prevention: a systematic review. Early Interv Psychiatry 10(2):103–121, 2016 25702826

Saberi P, Siedle-Khan R, Sheon N, et al: The use of mobile health applications among youth and young adults living with HIV: focus group findings. AIDS Patient Care STDs 30(6):254–260, 2016 27214751

Saha K, Torous J, Ernala SK, et al: A computational study of mental health awareness campaigns on social media. Transl Behav Med 9(6):1197–1207, 2019 30834942

Shah RN, Berry OO: The rise of venture capital investing in mental health. JAMA Psychiatry 78(4):351, 2020 32936238

Su C, Xu Z, Pathak J, et al: Deep learning in mental health outcome research: a scoping review. Transl Psychiatry 10(1):116, 2020 32532967

Thomas N, McLeod B, Jones N, et al: Developing internet interventions to target the individual impact of stigma in health conditions. Internet Interv 2(3):351–358, 2015

Thomas VL, Chavez M, Browne EN, et al: Instagram as a tool for study engagement and community building among adolescents: a social media pilot study. Digit Health 6:2055207620904548, 2020 32215216

Toombs E, Kowatch KR, Dalicandro L, et al: A systematic review of electronic mental health interventions for Indigenous youth: results and recommendations. J Telemed Telecare 27(9):539–552, 2021 31937199

Vogels EA, Gelles-Watnick R, Massarat N, et al: Teens, social media and technology 2022. Pew Research Center, August 10, 2022. Available at: https://

www.pewresearch.org/internet/2022/08/10/teens-social-media-and-technology-2022. Accessed December 6, 2023.

Wind TR, Rijkeboer M, Andersson G, et al: The COVID-19 pandemic: The "black swan" for mental health care and a turning point for e-health. Internet Interv 20:100317, 2020 32289019

Zhang R, Nicholas J, Knapp AA, et al: Clinically meaningful use of mental health apps and its effects on depression: mixed methods study. J Med Internet Res 21(12):e15644, 2019 31859682

Zheng Y, Walsham G: Inequality of what? An intersectional approach to digital inequality under COVID-19. Inf Organ 31(1):100341, 2021

14

Youth Agency, Rights, and the Promise of a Well-Designed Digital World

Amanda Third, Ph.D.

When children have agency and can make meaningful choices, both their motivation and their psychological health are more likely to flourish (Deci and Ryan 2000). But what does children's agency look like in relation to the digital environment? What can be done to enable it? In this chapter, I ask to what extent it is possible to develop digital products with children's agency and rights in mind, an idea contrary to historical practice. In search of an answer, I turn to children's own expertise about their rights in the digital environment, exploring how young people configure their agency in the digital world and what guidance they have that might aid the design of digital products, platforms, and services that respect their rights.

The perspectives of children laid out here draw on in-depth qualitative consultations with 709 children ages 10–18 years from 27 countries (Third and Moody 2021) to inform the drafting of the U.N. Committee on the Rights of the Child's (UNCRC; 2021) general comment No. 25 on children's rights in relation to the digital environment (GC25). Defining the *digital environment* as encompassing "information and communications technologies, including digital networks, content services, and applications, connected devices and environments, virtual and augmented reality, artificial intelligence, robotics, automated systems, algorithms and data analytics, biometrics and implant technology," this landmark guidance details how states should interpret the 30-plus year-old Convention on the Rights of the Child for the digital age (United Nations Committee on the Rights of the Child 2021).

In narrating children's insights, I have been concerned with reflecting accurately the ways children in the study articulated what they found enabling and disabling about the digital environment. However, I fully acknowledge that all such efforts to represent children's views are always already acts of translation and, consequently, are imperfect. What follows, then, is an intergenerational effort to articulate what is important to children about their agency in relation to the digital environment.

Child Rights, Agency, and the Design of the Digital Environment

Since at least 2014, when the UNCRC hosted a Day of General Discussion on children's rights and digital media (see Office of the United Nations Commissioner for Human Rights 2014), child rights approaches have progressively dominated digital policy, programming, and product design in many parts of the world for children younger than 18 years.

Child rights approaches to the digital environment are grounded in the UNCRC, a legally binding international agreement stipulating the civil, political, social, economic, and cultural rights to which all youth everywhere, regardless of race, ability, or religion, are entitled (Office of the United Nations High Commissioner for Human Rights 1989). Although the Convention makes no explicit mention of children's agency, a concept of the agentic child underpins its 54 articles. For example, the Convention enshrines children's rights to participation (see Lansdown 2010; United Nations Committee on the Rights of the Child 2009), calling youth into being as rights-claiming, agentic subjects. Article 12—the right to be heard—is recognized as one of the four guiding principles that drive the implementation of the Convention, alongside the child's right to life and survival (Article 6), the child's right to enjoy their rights without discrimination (Article 2), and the best interests of the child as the primary consideration (Article 3) (see Office of the United Nations High Commissioner for Human Rights 1989). Granting children a degree of self-determination, in accordance with their age and level of maturity—or evolving capacities (Article 5; see Lansdown 2005)—distinguishes the Convention from previous declarations of children's rights. Indeed, we might argue that its vision of the agentic child is so radical that it is surprising that this Convention is the most widely ratified human rights instrument in history. The United States is the sole remaining U.N. member state that has not ratified or formally accepted the UNCRC.

A key milestone in establishing children's rights as imperative in the digital environment was the UNCRC's adoption of GC25 in early 2021 (United Nations Committee on the Rights of the Child 2021). Adhering to the Convention's stipulation for youth participation, this human rights instrument provides principled and evidence-based guidance, grounded in extensive international consultations with youth, experts, and other key stakeholders, for interpreting and applying the Convention in a world increasingly touched—and even structured—by "the digital" (Third et al. 2019b, p. 380). GC25 lays out states' (i.e., ratifying and formally accepting nations') obligations to protect, respect, and fulfill children's rights regarding the digital environment and includes guidance with implications for youth, parents and caregivers, governments, civil society, and the private sector. Acknowledging that children's lives are impacted by the digital environment even when they do not have direct access to it, GC25 describes access to digital technology and the internet as a condition of possibility for youth's capacity to claim and exercise their rights in the modern world. Furthermore, it not only advocates for these rights to apply in digital spaces but also imagines how digital technology might be harnessed to facilitate the full range of children's rights across what adults often describe as "online and offline" spaces.

GC25 remains true to the Convention's vision of the agentic child, making explicit reference to children's agency. At the same time, it asserts the possibilities of design for mitigating the physical, social, and psychological risks of harm that youth encounter, as well as augmenting the opportunities and benefits they derive from their digital participation. GC25 is not unique in looking to design as a remedy for the shortcomings of children's experiences of the digital world. The internet was never developed with children in mind (Livingstone and Third 2017), and in order to address this oversight, governments and civil society organizations have advanced a series of "by design" initiatives, including Safety by Design (eSafety Commissioner 2022), Child Rights by Design (D4CR Association 2023; Digital Futures Commission 2023a; Hartung 2020), Privacy by Design (Cavoukian 2011), Secure by Design (U.K. Department for Science, Innovation and Technology 2019), Playful by Design (Digital Futures Commission 2023b), and Age-Appropriate Design (Information Commissioner's Office 2020). The "by design" movement calls on industry, government, and civil society to ensure that the design of digital products and services prioritizes youth's needs, entitlements, and aspirations; as Australia's eSafety Commissioner is known to say, "by design" is about baking users' rights into the design of technologies.

However, this embrace of design potentially sits at odds with the vision of the agentic child that is at the heart of the Convention and GC25. Design implies the ordering and streamlining of human experience in accordance with dominant cultural values. It aims to prevent particular actions or behaviors or to encourage ("nudge") some over others. If design targets a seamless experience, agency is often at its optimal when it confronts degrees of friction. If all digital spaces are designed to some degree (Livingstone and Pothong 2021), how can we be sure that the design of digital spaces does not overly constrain children's agency to claim their rights or fail to value the myriad ways they conceive and enact their agency? What would it entail to design the digital environment to foster children's agency? Is that even possible?

Children's Views on the Potential of Digital Environments to Augment Their Agency

What do youth's narrations of their digital practices tell us about how they understand agency in relation to the digital environment? Given the opportunity to speak about their digital practices, children worldwide tend to highlight the myriad ways that the digital environment supports and enhances their agency to explore, to learn and grow, and to realize their rights. Reflecting the way they imagine their online and face-to-face lives as integrated (Third et al. 2017), children indicate that their use of digital technology supports their agency to claim their rights in both online and offline spaces. Indeed, they have an expansive sense of how the digital enables them to claim the full range of their rights (all citations of children's views in this chapter are drawn from Third and Moody 2021).

> In the age of technology, if children learn to use the internet, they can be competitive in this life.
>
> —*male, Ethiopia, age 17*

> Having access to digital technology contributes to low unemployment rates, getting jobs, social justice, reaching out to others internationally, appreciating other cultures/differences.
>
> —*female, Canada, age 17*

In particular, children highlight the positive interlocking impacts of the digital environment on their relationships with family, peers, and others; education and learning; exploration of their identities; relaxation and play; expression; civic and political engagement on issues of importance to them; and their physical and mental health and well-being.

> Digital technology allows me to connect with friends and express myself in a safe environment.
>
> *—sex and age unknown, Pakistan*

> I can use my phone to search for information for school; I can see my grades online; I can watch content that can teach me a lot.
>
> *—female, Croatia, age 13*

> Digital technology introduced me to major aspects of how I identify myself, such as feminism and equal rights for all.
>
> *—female, Canada, age 15*

> You can study online if you are not capable of going to school.
>
> *—male, United Arab Emirates, age 16*

> The internet has brought us a huge diversity of activities for leisure and entertainment.
>
> *—female, Brazil, age 14*

> On the internet, I find more acceptance than in my "real life" surroundings, which showed me that it is okay to be different.
>
> *— female, Germany, age 16*

> The evolution of technology helps more and more people through the expansion of access [to health services].
>
> — *female, Romania, age 16*

> When you are sad, the internet can help you see something that brings you joy and makes you happier.
>
> —*male, Brazil, age 13*

Indeed, given the growing importance of the digital to everyday life in many places around the world, children say that access to digital technology and the internet is a precondition of their capacity to exercise their agency to claim and enact their rights. Some even believe that access to the internet should be a right in and of itself.

> To me, the internet is a right. It is the main means to communicate today.
>
> —*male, Brazil, age unknown*

We might describe the sense of agency in these statements as instrumental in that they have a trajectory (indicated by the preposition in "agency *to*"), are motivated by a means-ends dynamic, are accompanied by a strong degree of intentionality, and configure digital technology primarily as a tool children can wield to take action in ways that make sense to them. Alongside their expressions of instrumental agency, youth also gesture toward a more emergent—but equally important and sometimes simultaneous—sense of agency that plays out in the digital spaces they inhabit. Here, rather than having identifiable aims and a clear trajectory, children's agency assumes a more exploratory, opportunistic, and even accidental quality.

> Your exploration of digital technology...helps you find yourself and define your interest[s. It helps you know] your identity.
>
> —*sex and age unknown, Pakistan*

> With the help of the internet, you can carve your own personality.
>
> —*female, Romania, age 15*

Such agency is found in immersion in the digital environment; it entails a process of dwelling in and with different possibilities and of tactically (Third et al. 2019a) seizing opportunities to act amid the eventualities that present themselves. It is associated in particular with relaxation and play, which are known to have positive impacts on children's mental health and well-being. In this configuration of their agency, children view the technology less as a tool and more as an environment ripe for exploration.

Children's agency is steered by their desires and is propelled by mobility (e.g., scrolling, clicking, watching, liking, reacting, flipping from screen to screen, mobilizing across online and offline boundaries, and so on). It often takes expression in rapid-fire micro-decision-making. Cumulatively, these micro-expressions of agency produce a sense of the technology as an ally with which they partner to locate and enact their agency. We can hear this partnership model of technology use—this sense of "working with"—in, for example, their descriptions of how they interact with and "teach" platforms' recommendation algorithms.

> On Instagram, you show the algorithm that you want to see more of something by liking, sharing, watching it; you show the algorithm that you want to see less of something by blocking or reporting.
>
> —*female, Germany, age 16*

Those children with routine and reliable access to the internet and digital technology emphasize that the digital environment makes knowledge, information, and opportunities much more accessible to them and makes it significantly easier for them to complete tasks, pursue curiosities, learn about themselves, and share their views and ideas.

> The internet is a very important form of information and communication because it is easy to use and very accessible.
>
> —*female, Brazil, age 14*

> Expressing our opinion is very important, and it has a big impact when it comes to the digital age, because in just one click the world can know your opinion.
> —*male, Philippines, age unknown*

Because their everyday lives typically unfold against a backdrop of rules, authority figures, and institutions that profoundly constrain their mobility and discipline their actions and interactions, children generally express an acute sense that the digital environment multiplies the number and range of opportunities to explore and exercise their agency. Indeed, some say it quite literally opens up the world for them in ways that would not be possible without it.

> [With] digital technology…we can connect ourselves to the world and we can make an identity in the world.
> —*male, Pakistan, age 13*

> The digital environment creates equal opportunities; being without it limits quality of life.
> —*female, Canada, age 15*

Children note that the digital environment provides them with opportunities to experiment and develop skills, producing a mastery that in turn fuels their sense of agency. Many have a sense of pride, for example, in the expertise they have developed about technology and claim they can teach adults a thing or two.

> Children and adolescents nowadays know more about the internet than adults.
> —*male, Portugal, age 19*

> I could teach an adult how to use a more advanced phone or a smart device.
> —*female, Romania, age 14*

> I can teach adults about [the] games and search engines of today's generation.
>
> —*female, South Korea, age 12*

Across cultural contexts, young people configure their agency in relation to the digital environment in profoundly relational terms. They note that their relationships with parents and caregivers, friends, peers, and others provide them with the necessary encouragement and support to exercise their agency. For example, many children interviewed noted that parents and caregivers bolster their confidence and guide them in expressing themselves online.

> My parents show commitment to my online self-expression and think it's cool that youths are engaged.
>
> —*female, Norway, age 16*

> My parents support me so that I can be psychologically re-laxed and expressive…in the [online] community, but in a respectful way.
>
> —*female, Lebanon, age 16*

> Sometimes when we need help solving problems online, we ask parents to help us solve our questions or problems.
>
> —*group activity, Chile*

Children also find like-minded individuals and communities of interest in the digital environment, which supports them in exploring their worlds, exchanging information, and taking action either individually or collectively, including in relation to civil and political issues. This dimension of the digital environment's support for their agency appears to increase as they grow older.

> Access to social media helped me find [movements] I really agree with, i.e., feminism (#metoo) and climate change (#fridaysforthefuture).
>
> —*female, Canada, age 15*

> I use online threads to discuss important issues with others.
> —*female, Indonesia, age 14*

> I can find many people online with whom I share the same
> cultural identity...and we can encourage one another that
> it is okay to be ourselves.
> —*female, Canada, age 18*

Moreover, children highlight that the digital environment augments their agency in the here and now and will continue to do so into their futures.

> Technology is very important, and it will continue to be in
> the future. It is hard to communicate without it. Everything
> is here, on the cell phone. I can find information about al-
> most anything. I can talk to my friends whenever and wher-
> ever I want to. The world is moving forward, and so we
> must do the same.
> —*female, Croatia, age 12*

Overall, then, children paint a striking picture of the possibilities for their agency enabled by the digital environment. However, they are also very clear that they confront a range of significant barriers to their agency. It is to these dimensions of children's experiences as agentic subjects in the digital environment to which I now turn.

Agency Between Liberation and Constraint

Although young people experience moments of both fleeting and sustained agency in relation to the digital environment, they also routinely encounter breaches of and constraints on their agency when engaging online, often leading them to express frustration, disappointment, or anger. These sentiments are evident, for example, in the ways they narrate how the attitudes, behaviors, and limitations of adults in their lives impede their agency.

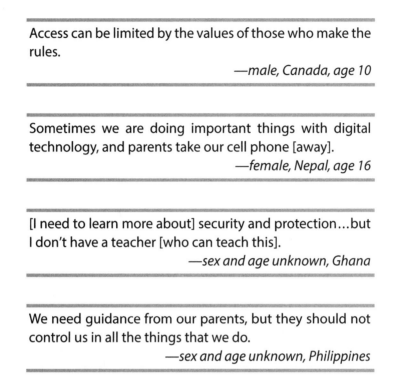

> Access can be limited by the values of those who make the rules.
>
> *—male, Canada, age 10*

> Sometimes we are doing important things with digital technology, and parents take our cell phone [away].
>
> *—female, Nepal, age 16*

> [I need to learn more about] security and protection…but I don't have a teacher [who can teach this].
>
> *—sex and age unknown, Ghana*

> We need guidance from our parents, but they should not control us in all the things that we do.
>
> *—sex and age unknown, Philippines*

Indicating how their agency to claim their rights is deeply grounded in and often limited by socio-material factors, children also report that a range of challenges prevent their routine and reliable access to the internet and to digital devices, thereby constraining their agency. These include poor electricity, unreliable connectivity, the cost of devices and data, and their reliance on old devices or those shared among family members.

> We don't express ourselves using digital technologies as much as we would like to…because we don't have smartphones because of financial constraints.
>
> *—sex and age unknown, Pakistan*

> I am sincerely hoping that the signals in rural areas can be strengthened and the financial problems will be overcome.
>
> *—female, Malaysia, age 13*

> [There is] no power in our area.
>
> *—male, Kenya, age 15*

Some children also note that the lack of online content in a language they speak is a major barrier to their capacity to use the internet to exercise their agency as rights-holding individuals.

> Crioulo [Portuguese Creole], my main language, is never on the internet.
>
> *—male, Portugal, age 13*

Clearly, more needs to be done to improve access to digital technologies for children around the world, particularly in the global South. At the same time, those instances when their capacity to act is minimized or thwarted are formative for children's conception of their agency in relation to the digital environment. Children come to know their agency in part through its limits. Additionally, confronting obstacles can produce in children the impetus to marshal their agency to find effective work arounds, thereby identifying new forms of agency for themselves.

Indeed, to the extent that agency is an imagined capacity, we might say that children's sense of it emerges from the interplay between the more liberatory impulses they associate with the digital environment and the (sometimes quite significant) constraints they experience therein. To illustrate this point, I give three short examples of this double movement shaping how children imagine their agency.

Information

Children say that the digital environment gives them access to vast amounts of knowledge and information that would not otherwise be available to them, facilitating their agency to explore their worlds and their identities, participate in their communities, and support their well-being. They report, for example, that the opportunity to find information about taboo or sensitive topics in the digital environment, such as mental health and sexual and reproductive health, grants them a form of agency that they cannot find elsewhere. This agency, which originates online, extends into and has an impact on their face-to-face worlds.

I learned how to clean up my body after menstruation, based on my religion.

—female, Indonesia, age unknown

I [asked] about things I felt ashamed to ask Mom about—different woman things—and the internet helped me.

—female, Russia, age unknown

I researched about mental illness, depression, and anxiety out of curiosity, because nobody talked about it and I wanted to know more.

—male, Brazil, age 14

Indeed, some children underscore that the information they access in the digital environment has a protective value for them. Here, we might note that children's agency often assumes a defensive quality; it is exercised precisely to protect themselves.

Access to information [online] is important so you don't get exploited by others.

—female, Norway, age 17

The right to information is…important in the digital age because it helps us to access information easier. But we need to keep in mind that not all information on social media is true and reliable. Wrong information can influence a child and cause her/him harm.

—male, Philippines, age unknown

As technology grows, we can easily access information. But it's hard to know whether the information is valid or not.

—female, Indonesia, age 14

In relation to their right to information, then, children's sense of agency emerges along a spectrum between ideas about the unlimited informational potential of the digital environment and the knowledge that not all information is trustworthy. In this sense, giving children opportunities to explore diverse sources of information and to refine their critical sensibilities will be vital to enabling their agency in relation to their right to information.

Data, Privacy, and Exploitation

When it comes to data, the double movement shaping children's agency plays out in a tension between access to free services and the potential for exploitation. Many children are confident that they have agency over the management of their privacy and can minimize their exposure to potential harms caused by the movement of their data across proprietary platforms.

> I can control who will see my information [on] social media and who will not. I can choose who will see my posts, images, and information [on] my account, and I can choose who will not.
>
> —*female, Philippines, age unknown*

> I don't have/put anything I don't want on the internet on my social media. But when I do it's blocked from others that I don't want to see it.
>
> —*male, Canada, age 15*

In fact, many children—especially those in the global North—are cognizant that the current business models of platforms and products grant them free access to platforms in exchange for their data.

> Apps collect...your data. They sell this. You know you are exposed, because you get ads.
>
> —*female, Norway, age 17*

> If the social media platforms didn't sell data, then they wouldn't be able to function.
> —*male, United Kingdom, age 17*

> Social media is free because you are the product, meaning they can sell your data to advertisers and different companies without you knowing.
> —*female, Canada, age 14*

Some children say they believe this is a fair price to pay to be able to connect with peers and family and have access to unlimited information. However, many more are less convinced that this is a fair exchange.

> Digital rights are human rights. It shouldn't be a trade.
> —*female, United Kingdom, age 17*

> It's never a fair trade for your personal information. These platforms sell information to other companies, therefore it's always important to keep…certain information [to yourself].
> —*female, Canada, age 13*

Children's sense that such pacts with companies are exploitative and compromise their agency is all the more acute because the terms of engagement with platforms are not always explicit to them, wrapped up, as they are, in impenetrable terms and conditions.

> Generally, it is a gigantic riddle what happens to our data, as it is hidden in complex data protection agreements and legal texts. I would like to obtain clarity about what really happens with my data.
> —*female, Germany, age 16*

> I want to be told where the information I enter into web-sites goes. I also want to know which people have access to that information and can I be sure that they'll keep it private.
>
> —*female, Philippines, age unknown*

Some children draw attention to the asymmetrical power relationships and coercive dynamics at the heart of their interactions with proprietary platforms—namely, that they have little choice but to accept companies' terms wholesale if they wish to engage with their family, peer, and interest-based networks.

> [Social media platforms] are known for spreading/gathering personal data, but due to social obligations and pressures, I do not plan to stop using these platforms.
>
> —*female, Canada, age 18*

In their renderings of these dynamics, youth implicitly acknowledge that their agency fluctuates according to different time scales. In the short term, they can choose to exchange their data for access to free platforms and services, and this facilitates their immediate agency, for example, to connect with others and seek out information. Nonetheless, they recognize that, in the long term, exercising this agency may not serve their interests and, indeed, may reduce their agency over their data into the future. There is significant scope, here, for technology platforms to deploy strategies, such as offering users generative artificial intelligence to explore terms and conditions before signing up to platforms, enabling them to exercise more agency over their data and privacy and to protect themselves from exploitation.

Identity and Expression

Children report that engaging with the digital environment offers them opportunities to express their ideas and opinions and, thereby, to explore their identities. In their descriptions of the value they place on expression, we can detect strong overtones of their agentic selves.

> I like writing stories, poetry, and memoirs and sharing them online for anyone from friends to strangers to read.

> Having a place to digitally explore my writing motivates me to write more, helps me feel organized, and gets my ideas and stories out in the world.
>
> —*female, Canada, age 17*

> By writing posts, I share my point of view regarding feminism because more people will read it, as everyone uses social media.
>
> —*sex and age unknown, Pakistan*

Although they value the expressive potentialities of the digital environment, they also worry that sharing their views will unduly expose them to the negative judgments of others, with consequences for their mental health and well-being. Underscoring the relational dimensions that proscribe children's agency in the digital environment, some note that their agency to express themselves is tempered by the potentially negative reactions of others. Some discussed how they exercise agency through self-censorship.

> On the internet, we're more susceptible to people judging our thoughts and opinions, which makes it harder for us to have freedom of expression. We tend to suppress our thoughts in order to fit ourselves in a mold in order to not be judged by the internet.
>
> —*sex and age unknown, New Zealand*

> I'm just too…nervous to voice out my opinion.
>
> —*female, Canada, age 12*

> I don't express myself out of fear of being bullied.
>
> —*female, Germany, age 18*

Here, in children's reluctance to exercise their right to expression, we can see how the exercise of agency sometimes takes a defensive posture, often demanding both vigilance and resilience. In this sense, children's agency is not straightforwardly unproblematic. Indeed, children themselves are quick to acknowledge that there are limits to their agency. Many say that they need to exercise their agency with care for others.

> I take into account minorities and those people who may be personally affected before posting controversial information.
>
> —*male, Pakistan, age 16*

Clearly, much could be done to ensure that online spaces better protect children when they exercise their agency to express themselves.

The double movement implicit in these examples of how children call their agency into being reminds us that, although they remain optimistic about the opportunities of the digital environment, as subordinate subjects, children navigate power relations and significant limits on their agency on multiple fronts. Theirs is always already a subaltern agency seeking opportunities to escape constraint. When such opportunities present in and across the digital environment, children are seizing them to reinvent agency in interesting and potentially world-changing ways.

Reinventing Agency:
From Individual Action to Collective Activism

In this chapter I have traced how, from children's perspectives, the digital environment accentuates both the limits and the possibilities for children to exercise their agency. However, beyond an escalation of the dynamics that shape their agency in the face-to-face world, what is unique about the ways in which the digital environment enables or constrains it? To answer this question, let us turn to children's framings of their civic and political agency.

Throughout the consultations, children around the world drew attention to how the digital environment augments their agency to learn about and contribute to social and political change. Indeed, children appear to see the internet as a game-changer for social movements internationally.

> Social justice plays a huge role in social change, and the internet is the biggest platform to advocate for social justice. This way, everyone has a voice.
>
> —*female, Canada, age 18*

Many children are already using the digital environment to take action on issues they care about, and many others express a desire to step up their efforts to do so.

> Digital technology enables me to learn about the environmental issues that take place around the world, which is something I find important. This is how social media helps grow my identity.
>
> —*female, Canada, age 15*

> I would like to take more action online.
>
> —*female, Pakistan, age 12*

> I would like to use digital technologies to improve the world, which I don't really do now. I would nonetheless like to do it as it would be something positive and serve the general good.
>
> —*male, Germany, age 16*

Given the tendency for contemporary cultures to construct children as enthusiastic adopters of technology, it perhaps seems commonsensical that children would be passionate about the potential of digital technology to supercharge social and political change. But why are they so convinced of its power to deliver transformation? Explaining this requires a brief diversion.

In his 1983 book *Imagined Communities: Reflections on the Origins and Spread of Nationalism*, Benedict Anderson coined the term "imagined communities" to explain how large communities, in which it is impossible for all members to meet face-to-face, constitute themselves as national communities by imagining their belonging to the nation-state. Anderson was interested in the ways that the rise of nationalism, as the characteristic political assemblage of modernity, coincided with the introduction and widespread uptake of the mechanical printing press, the spread of print capitalism, and the capacity to distribute printed materials at scale in what became "mass media." For Anderson, the private act of sitting down to read the national newspaper each morning at the same time as others was an important mechanism by which people imagined themselves as members of the nation, thereby helping to call the very idea of the nation into being.

It is worth thinking through the significance of Anderson's imagined communities in relation to the digital environment. Of course, interfacing with digital media is not the same as reading a newspaper; for example, online information flows are multidirectional and asynchronous. Nonetheless, the digital environment enables youth, as a subordinate group, to connect with each other, share information, and organize, offering them an unprecedented possibility to imagine themselves as a global political constituency with the agency to call for and enact widespread social change. For the first time in history, children's sense of unity with other children can extend well beyond their local communities. They can find each other and establish solidarity across international borders. We are already seeing the power of this identity formation manifest, for example, in hundreds of thousands of children around the world using their smartphones and tablets to organize and take to the streets to call for climate justice as part of the "Fridays for the Future" student protests. Imagine if this form of collective agency could be amplified. Imagine, too, the effect this empowerment and sense of agency could have on the well-being of a generation of youth.

Conclusion

In this chapter, I have traced the ways that children narrate their agency in relation to the digital environment. By way of conclusion, I return to the question of what it might mean to design products for children's agency. Reading their insights about the digital world, it is clear that children have sophisticated understandings of how their agency is both constrained and enabled in relation to the digital environment. In turn, if it is indeed possible to design the digital environment to foster children's agency, there can be no one-size-fits-all solution. Rather, the task is to acknowledge and design with the diversity of children's experiences in mind. As I have shown, agency unfolds across diverse scales. It has both short- and long-term dimensions, and it may take either more instrumental or more emergent forms. Youth might, at different moments or simultaneously, imagine their agency in individual or collective ways. Their conceptions of and capacities to exercise it will change according to their trajectories of growth and development. Children's agency is profoundly shaped by the very diverse cultural and socio-material contexts that shape their face-to-face lives in different places in the world, and although we might have some understanding of how it presently operates in relation to the digital environment, how it materializes likely will continue to mutate into the future as the digital environment itself evolves.

Given this, the task of designing for all possible potentialities is deeply challenging, if not impossible. Here, it is useful to search first for a metaphor, and then for a set of practical strategies, to guide our approach to respecting, protecting, and fulfilling children's agency to claim their rights in the digital age. For the former, we might consider Donald Winnicott's concept of a "holding space," an emotional and physical environment in which the child can gradually transition from absolute dependence on the mother to becoming "a self-experiencing being" (Winnicott 1987, p. 7). Underpinned by a fundamentally agentic theorization of the child, Winnicott's idea of the holding space enables the growing child, over time, to venture farther and farther away along a radius from the mother, to explore their world but always with the possibility of looking back to the mother for her reassurance. The holding space is safe but imperfect and uncomfortable, a learning space that is supportive but oriented to curiosity, risk, and, ultimately, independence. It is a space with flexible boundaries that extend as the child learns to find their way in the world. Could user experience and other designers of social digital environments create digital holding spaces intentionally designed to "mature" as their users do? Could artificial intelligence be used to design deep "learning spaces" online or spaces tailored to change with kids to the specifications of educators, parents, and caregivers?

Whatever metaphor we use, we will be unable to design safe, healthy, and stimulating spaces without listening carefully to the people that they are intended to serve. We need to understand and take seriously children's suggestions about how to build digital environments in which they can find, experiment with, and enact their agency in ways that not only meet their needs but fulfill the full range of their rights, as stipulated by the UNCRC. It is perhaps fitting that a child has the last say:

> When governments [and others] are making decisions, they must talk with…children to know if children are comfortable or not in that decision. Decisions [about children's lives] shouldn't be conducted…without children's participation. All children are equals.
>
> —*female, Nepal, age 16*

References

Anderson B: Imagined Communities: Reflections on the Origins and Spread of Nationalism. London, Verso, 1983

Cavoukian A: Privacy by Design: The 7 Foundational Principles. Toronto, ON, Canada, Information and Privacy Commissioner, 2011. Available at: https://iapp.org/media/pdf/resource_center/pbd_implement_7found_principles.pdf. Accessed May 1, 2023.

Deci EL, Ryan RM: The "what" and "why" of goal pursuits: human needs and the self-determination of behavior. Psychol Inq 11(4):227–268, 2000

D4CR Association: Designing for Children's Rights: Integrating Children's Rights Into Design and Business. D4CR, 2023. Available at: http://designingforchildrensrights.org. Accessed May 1, 2023.

Digital Futures Commission: Child Rights by Design Toolkit. London, Digital Futures Commission, 2023a. Available at: https://digitalfuturescommission.org.uk/wp-content/uploads/2023/03/CRbD_report-FINAL-Online.pdf. Accessed May 1, 2023.

Digital Futures Commission: Playful by Design Toolkit. London, Digital Futures Commission, 2023b. Available at: https://digitalfuturescommission.org.uk/playful-by-design-toolkit/. Accessed May 1, 2023.

eSafety Commissioner: Safety by design. Sydney, Australian Government, 2022. Available at: https://www.esafety.gov.au/industry/safety-by-design. Accessed January 25, 2023.

Hartung P: The Children's Rights-by-Design Standard for Data Use by Tech Companies. Good Governance of Children's Data Project, No 5. New York, UNICEF Office of Global Insight and Policy, 2020. Available at: https://www.unicef.org/globalinsight/media/1286/file/%20UNICEF-Global-Insight-DataGov-data-use-brief-2020.pdf. Accessed May 1, 2023.

Information Commissioner's Office: Age Appropriate Design: A Code of Practice for Online Services. United Kingdom, Information Commissioner's Office, 2020. Available at: https://ico.org.uk/media/for-organisations/guide-to-data-protection/key-data-protection-themes/age-appropriate-design-a-code-of-practice-for-online-services-2-1.pdf. Accessed May 1, 2023.

Lansdown G: The Evolving Capacities of the Child. New York, Innocenti Insights, UNICEF Office of Research, No 11. 2005. Available at: https://www.unicef-irc.org/publications/384-the-evolving-capacities-of-the-child.html. Accessed May 1, 2023.

Lansdown G: The realisation of children's participation rights: critical reflections, in A Handbook of Children and Young People's Participation: Perspectives From Theory and Practice. Edited by Percey-Smith B, Thomas N. New York, Routledge, 2010, pp 11–23

Livingstone S, Pothong K: What Is Meant by "By Design"? Playful By Design: A Vision of Free Play in the Digital World. London, Digital Futures Commission and 5Rights Foundation, November 2021. Available at: https://digitalfuturescommission.org.uk/wp-content/uploads/2021/11/A-Vision-of-Free-Play-in-a-Digital-World.pdf. Accessed December 6, 2023.

Livingstone S, Third A: Children and young people's rights in the digital age: an emerging agenda. New Media Soc 19(5):657–670, 2017

Office of the United Nations High Commissioner for Human Rights: Convention on the Rights of the Child. New York, United Nations, 1989. Available at: https://www.ohchr.org/en/instruments-mechanisms/instruments/convention-rights-child. Accessed May 1, 2023.

Office of the United Nations High Commissioner for Human Rights: 2014 Day of General Discussion: Digital Media and Children's Rights. Geneva, Office of the United Nations High Commissioner for Human Rights, 2014. Available at: https://www.ohchr.org/en/events/days-general-discussion-dgd/2014/2014-day-general-discussion-digital-media-and-childrens. Accessed April 2024.

Third A, Moody L: Our Rights in the Digital World: A Report on the Children's Consultations to Inform UNCRC General Comment 25. London, 5Rights Foundation and Western Sydney University, 2021. Available at: https://www.westernsydney.edu.au/__data/assets/pdf_file/0011/1845497/Our_Rights_in_a_Digital_World_-_Full_Report.pdf. Accessed May 1, 2023.

Third A, Bellerose D, De Oliveira JD, et al: Young and Online: Children's Perspectives on Life in the Digital Age: The State of the World's Children 2017 Companion Report. New York, Institute for Culture and Society, UNICEF, 2017. Available at: https://www.westernsydney.edu.au/__data/assets/pdf_file/0006/1334805/Young_and_Online_Report.pdf. Accessed December 6, 2023.

Third A, Collin P, Walsh L, et al: Young People in Digital Society: Control Shift. London, Palgrave Macmillan, 2019a

Third A, Livingstone S, Lansdown G: Recognizing children's rights in relation to digital technologies: challenges of voice and evidence, principle, and practice, in Research Handbook on Human Rights and Digital Technology. Edited by Wagner B, Kettemann MC, Vieth K. Northampton, MA, Edward Elgar Publishing, 2019b, pp 376–410

U.K. Department for Science, Innovation and Technology: Secure by Design. Gov.uk, 2019. Available at: https://www.gov.uk/government/collections/secure-by-design. Accessed May 1, 2023.

United Nations Committee on the Rights of the Child: General comment No. 12 on right of the child to be heard (CRC/C/GC/12). New York, United Nations, July 20, 2009. Available at: https://digitallibrary.un.org/record/671444/files/CRC_C_GC_12-EN.pdf. Accessed May 1, 2023.

United Nations Committee on the Rights of the Child: General Comment No. 25 on Children's Rights in Relation to the Digital Environment (CRC/C/GC/25). New York, United Nations, March 2, 2021. Available at: https://www.ohchr.org/en/documents/general-comments-and-recommendations/general-comment-no-25-2021-childrens-rights-relation. Accessed May 1, 2023.

Winnicott WD: The ordinary devoted mother, in Babies and Their Mothers. Reading, MA, Addison-Wesley, 1987, p 7

Index

Page numbers printed in **boldface** type refer to figures and tables.